DR. SHINTANI'S
EAT MORE,
Weigh Less ™
DIET

Terry Shintani, M.D., J.D., M.P.H.

Halpax

HP

Composition and cover design by Halpax Publishing
Illustration by Terry Shintani, M.D., J.D., M.P.H., Dover
Publishing, and Avery Publishing Group Inc. (Garden City
Park, N.Y.). *Changing Seasons Macrobiotic Cookbook* by
Aveline Kushi and Wendy Esko, used by permission.

ISBN 0-9636117-0-4

1st printing, April 1993
2nd printing, September 1993, Revised
3rd printing, January 1994

10 9 8 7 6 5 4 3

Manufactured in the United States of America

Dedication

I would like to dedicate this book to the memory of my parents, Robert and Emi Shintani who taught me the values that have made me what I am today, and who, if they were alive, would have been amused that I named the "EMI" scale in this book after Mom.

Acknowledgements

Producing any book requires the effort of many people. I would like to acknowledge the assistance of the following people who have contributed to the creation of this book. I would like to thank Ms. J.M.T. Miller, a talented writer who helped me write the manuscript and Mr. Ray Brosseau for his brilliant editing of the book. Thanks also go to Sheila Beckham, M.P.H., R.D., C.D.E. and Joda Derrickson, M.P.H., R.D. who helped to review the recipes and nutrition information in the book, and Nadine Bruce, M.D. who reviewed the manuscript. Kathy Cain, R.N. helped me to compile the recipes, and Ms. Ann Tang and Ms. Elaine French contributed additional recipes. Ruth Heidrich, M.S. a world class triathlete and co-host of my nutrition radio talk-show reviewed the exercise portion of the book. I would also like to acknowledge my assistant, Mr. Jack Ke`ali`i Ha`o, whose tireless effort has helped make this book a reality.

Before You Change Your Diet and Exercise Level

Do NOT change your diet or exercise level without guidance from your medical doctor if you have health problems or are on medication. Do NOT change your medications without the guidance of your medical doctor. The information in this book is general information about your health and is NOT to be taken as professional advice or serve as a substitute for medical attention. The advice in this book is directed toward reasonably healthy adults. Individual needs do vary and for those with special conditions or needs, for children and pregnant women, modifications may be necessary and should be made under guidance of your medical doctor or registered dietitian.

TABLE OF CONTENTS

2

Part III Stay Healthy with the Eat More, Weigh Less Diet

Bibliography   272

PREFACE

Can eating MORE cause you to lose weight and even change your life? You bet it can. In 1976, as a first year law student, I changed my diet. I didn't do it to lose weight (I was only a little overweight). I didn't do it to cure an illness (I had no serious illness). But I was tired all the time, and was having trouble keeping up with the demands of law school. A friend suggested that my problem might be caused by the junk foods I was eating. I was skeptical, but nothing else was working so I decided to change my eating habits. It actually <u>did</u> change my life.

The transformation in me was astonishing, and happened almost overnight. I had more energy than ever before in my life, my thought processes became crystal clear, my grades improved and I published in the law review. I also (incidentally) lost 35 pounds in four months and felt better than ever before in my whole life. But as astonishing as all this may seem, the thing that really astounded me was that I did this while EATING MORE FOOD than ever before!

I was so stunned by the improvement in my health and the quality of my life that I wondered why nobody, physicians included, had ever told me diet could have such a dramatic impact. I wanted to understand what had happened to me, so I began researching everything I could find on the subject. There was a lot of research indicating health could be improved dramatically and that many of the major illnesses could be prevented and even reversed by a change in diet. I was again astonished to learn that in spite of this information, most Americans were then, and still are, dying from diet-related disease, and that most physicians did not know about or use diet much in the treatment of these diseases.

As a result of my experience and the new knowledge I had gained, I changed my career. I decided to become a physician and to learn as much as possible about using diet as a way to prevent and treat disease and obesity. Because we learned so little in medical school about nutrition, I went on to Harvard University to learn as much as I could about nutrition. I also became determined to spread the word to as many people as possible. I am convinced that a change in diet is the key to solving many of our health problems, our crisis in health care costs, and even many of humanity's problems in general.

I now use nutrition for both prevention of and intervention in disease. I have tried to learn all I can about ancient and non-industrialized cultures and their traditional diets, because the obesity and illnesses that plague modern American society were and are rare in ancient times and modern cultures which still follow their traditional diets. Ancient societies had people who were slim and full of vitality, creativity, and health. I believe that by returning to this type of diet and the lifestyle principles of our ancestors, we can regain our health without constantly resorting to medication. I also believe that diet is the key to maximizing our performance and our quality of life. This book will show you how to achieve these goals. It will also help you achieve natural weight loss while EATING MORE food. And it will show you not only how to minimize disease, but also how to maximize your health.

The approach you're about to learn works for most people. My own patients have proven that to me, time and again. And I and my colleagues have published a paper about the effectiveness of this approach. In fact, this diet is so effective that those who have health problems must see a physician before beginning the program, in order to get medical approval. Otherwise, the sudden change to your system might cause problems for you.

This book is yet another way for me to share the vital information that I first learned as a law student, and developed in medical school and in my studies in the field of nutrition. I hope that this information may motivate you to also change your diet so that you can learn to "Eat More, Weigh Less" and even change your life just as it did for me many years ago.

With much Aloha

Terry Shintani, MD, JD, MPH
Honolulu, 1993

INTRODUCTION

Congratulations! By picking up this book, you have identified yourself as someone who is interested in your health and is willing to do something about it. You are about to read about a revolutionary concept in weight loss.

Are you tired of dieting? If you are, this book may be what you're looking for. Recent studies have shown that most diets really don't work and can even be harmful. (1,2) This book turns the traditional concept of dieting upside down and replaces these old ideas with a healthy plan for weight loss designed around the latest research - a plan that can be sustained for the rest of your life.

Here are some of the startling things you will learn in this book.

- How to lose weight while eating up to 200% MORE FOOD

- A revolutionary way to find foods that will promote weight loss

- Why, in the long run, it's better to eat MORE to weigh less

- Five great myths about dieting in America

- How to lose weight while you sleep

- The one category of food to avoid for easy weight loss

- How to make your hunger work for you instead of against you

- Six steps to lower your cholesterol in just 30 days

- How to avoid 6 of the 10 leading causes of death in the United States

- How to prepare easy weight loss foods

WHAT THE DIET IS NOT

The Eat More, Weigh Less Diet is **not a "fad diet"**. Actually, it is **not even a "diet"** in the usual sense because there is **no calorie counting**. There are no powders, pills or magic bullets. It is not a diet which depends on portion control, and you won't need to exercise impossible self discipline. There are no gimmicks in the Eat More Diet program, and you're going to get slim and stay slim by using real food. It's a brand new up-to-the-minute scientifically supported plan that has worked for real people in real life situations, and this book will show you how it can work for you.

WHY THE "EAT MORE, WEIGH LESS" DIET?

It's called the "Eat More, Weigh Less" Diet because, as strange as it sounds, much of the recent research on obesity actually shows that you can lose weight by eating more. I've also called this book the "Eat More, Weigh Less" Diet because, frankly, I wanted to get your attention. Believe it or not, however, I do intend to show you how to Eat More and Weigh Less.

WHAT IS THE "EAT MORE, WEIGH LESS" DIET

Most diets tell you what not to do. The Eat More, Weigh Less Diet (usually referred to in this book as "Eat More Diet")tells you what you CAN do. The Eat More Diet program is deliberately designed so that it will not be a grueling exercise in self denial. Instead of teaching you how to do without food, the Eat More Diet will teach you how to EAT MORE and STILL LOSE WEIGHT. And, as a tremendous bonus, you'll probably lower your cholesterol level in under 30 days, possibly get rid of the need for some medications, and you will otherwise probably become healthier than you've ever been in your life.

The Eat More Diet is a new approach to weight loss that uses a collection of principles, techniques, tools, and recipes to help you to maximize your health. I have used them with great success in my practice and demonstrated the effectiveness of its underlying principle in a research project published in the American Journal of Clinical Nutrition. (3) I have developed five techniques and seven tools along with recipes and suggestions for your convenience.

TECHNIQUES

The Eat More Diet focuses on five main techniques:
1. How to "Eat More, Weigh Less" by choosing foods that satisfy your hunger while promoting weight loss (Chapter 3)
2. How to avoid foods that can increase body fat (Chapter 4)
3. Three ways to help you lose weight in your sleep (Chapter 5)
4. How to balance your diet (Chapter 7)
5. How to incorporate this diet into your lifestyle (Chapter 6)

TOOLS

The seven tools that I find most useful are:
1. A chart that I call the "Eat More Index" which helps you by indicating what foods will satisfy you the most, and what foods have the most fat in them.
2. The "Fat Finder Formula" which helps you find hidden fat in food
3. The Fat Gram approach to help limit the fat in your diet
4. A menu with recipes to show you how to prepare the food
5. The "Inverted Food Pyramid" which helps you balance your diet

6. A "Slim Pie" chart which is another diagram to
   help balance your diet
7. Additional diagrams and charts to show you
   how to make the Eat More Diet work for you.

HOW THIS BOOK IS ORGANIZED

This book is organized into three parts. The first part explains the principles behind the diet. The second part describes the diet and how to implement the diet including recipes and menus. The third part provides discusses special topics on diet and its impact on health.

WHY I DEVELOPED THE EAT MORE, WEIGH LESS DIET

The Eat More, Weigh Less Diet is actually a nutrition re-training program to help you maximize your health. I developed the program because, according to current statistics, nearly 70% of us are dying from diet-related diseases and being overweight is a major sign of this ongoing disaster. It made sense to me that the best way to treat any diet-related illness is to place people on a diet that duplicates the diets of people who rarely suffer from these diseases and are slim and healthy. It also turns out that these types of diets include foods which have an important quality about them that causes weight loss that we lack in our modern diets. In the Eat More Diet, I provide you with a simple way to find and use foods that have this quality in them which I call the "Eat More Index" (EMI).

WHAT IS THE "EAT MORE INDEX" (EMI)

I'll explain the EMI fully in a later chapter, but let me give you a preview of this index which I devised to help you examine which foods satisfy you the most per calorie. It is a totally new way of looking at food. The EMI number generally represents the number of pounds of food it takes to provide 2,500 calories or one day's worth of calories for an average active woman or average inactive man. For example, the EMI of corn is 6.1 which means that it takes 6.1 pounds of corn to make your daily calories. Obviously, you will have great difficulty eating this much corn and an easier time losing weight with such foods because it will fill your stomach before you get the

CAUSES OF DEATH
Ten Leading Causes
of Death in the U.S.

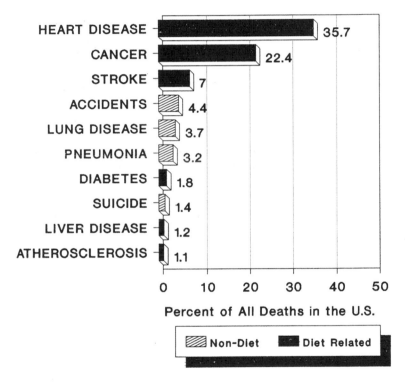

National Center for Health Statistics
1988

number of calories that would cause weight gain. Thus, the higher the EMI number of a food, that is, the more pounds of food it takes to provide your daily calories, the more likely you are to be satisfied by eating a selected food. Choosing foods in this way emphasizes the positive aspect of food and encourages people to "eat more" of these foods and helps promote automatic weight loss.

GETTING TO THE CAUSE OF OBESITY AND DISEASE

Using this approach, I have in my private practice reversed many illnesses and helped many people reduce or stop their dependence on various medications. The weight loss is incidental — a by-product of a healthy diet. If you follow the diet, the weight loss is automatic for most people if you are overweight. The reason I focus on weight loss is because being overweight is an early sign of poor health, and I want as many people as possible to avoid illness and the need for medication. I'd like to see as many people as possible to live a long and healthy life and avoid premature death. If you follow the proven program spelled out in this book, you, too, can enjoy all the rewards that come with being trim and in optimal health.

So—this book will provide a totally new, yet totally scientific perspective on weight loss. Some of this information may surprise you and the adjustments may not be easy. You will be rewarded for your effort by developing a fresh understanding of obesity, health, and disease, and you'll learn how to make it work for you. I want to teach you how to lose weight naturally. And by so doing, I am merely passing along a message from nature: obesity, disease, and less-than-optimal performance is nature's way of telling you that something is wrong with your diet! ESCAPE THE EPIDEMIC!

Make no mistake about it, we all need to learn to eat right! Almost a million Americans die every year from heart and vascular disease. One out of three people gets some form of cancer. There are countless other health problems, and most of them are sending us identical messages: we are suffering the consequences of a dietary epidemic. And obesity is just the tip of the iceberg. In fact, at present, nearly three out of every four people die from diet-related disease.

It is my fervent hope and prayer that this book will teach you what you need to know to escape the fate of the millions of people who are suffering because of improper diets. Because if you are like most people, you are literally eating yourself to death! In fact, the former Surgeon General, C. Everett Koop, warned us that in these United States the most common cause of death is—food! Being overweight is just an early sign of this far deeper problem. (5,6)

A SOLUTION

So what's the solution to this? You're on the right track by trying the Eat More Diet. All you need to do is take everything you learn to heart, realize that your very life may depend on what you learn in the Eat More Diet program, and then you can take the first positive steps toward increased health, longer life, and a trimmer and happier you. (7)

Thank you for reading this book and for looking after your health. I think you'll enjoy yourself with this book. After reading it, I hope you will commit yourself to trying the program for at least 14 days, or even better, use the principles for the rest of your life. You will learn how to be healthy and how to be ill. You will learn what foods cause you to be slim and what foods cause you to be overweight. Once you learn these things, the choice is yours.

MAKE THIS BOOK YOUR FRIEND

Now—please take a few more seconds to make this book your own. It's about you, it is for you. Like food itself, it can be your friend and your servant, so use it in any way that is helpful to you.

In fact, with regard to the principles in this book, you are what's important. You're more important than the ever-so-svelte model who's pushing 10,000 calorie hamburgers on TV and implying that without one you'll never be socially acceptable (she never eats them!); you're far more important than the waiter who looks down his nose because you're only ordering a salad. You're more important than all those friends who exert peer pressure to get you to help them devour a pizza, and you're even more important—for these purposes—than those members of your family who exert that subtle and not-so-subtle pressure on you to return to your old ways of eating. It's your body; it's your life. And this is your book, designed especially to help you maximize both your body's abilities and aesthetics, so that you can enjoy your life to the maximum! So—if you haven't already done so, please stop now and write your name on the inside cover, then fill in your name on the following certificate.

Certificate Of Value

This Eat More Diet Book is for

_____,

A Very Important Person

Now this book and the knowledge in it is yours.
Please use it to help change your life.

PART I

What to Do

CHAPTER 1

Eat Yourself Slim: The Basic Concept of the Eat More Diet

YOU REALLY CAN EAT MORE AND WEIGH LESS!

What if you could eat your way to a slim new you? Sound too good to be true? Of course it does. But the field of nutrition is finding that it can be true for you. And I'm delighted that you've given me the opportunity to be able to tell you exactly how to do it. Welcome to the Eat More, Weigh Less Diet.

If you're like most people who struggle to control their weight, you must be tired of others telling you that you need to eat less—especially if you're striving to do just that. Now you can happily inform these misguided critics that a better way to lose weight is to EAT MORE!

No joke!

Shocking though it may seem, eating more actually CAN make you lose weight - if you know how. Scientific evidence recently published in many of the most reputable journals in the world indicates that most of us are overweight in large part because we aren't eating enough of the kinds of foods that satisfies our hunger. This leaves us empty and craving more food, so we try to satisfy the resulting hunger by stuffing ourselves with the wrong kinds of food, and we end up overweight.

YOU'LL LOOK AT FOODS DIFFERENTLY!

I realize that the Eat More Diet concept runs counter to everything else you've ever learned about weight control. To make this program work for you, you'll have to learn to look at food in a totally different way. No more deliberate starving, no more counting calories, no more tiny portions and self denial. You'll learn how to choose foods based not on calories but on the "Eat More Index" (EMI) of Food, a unique way to discover what foods help you lose weight. The index grades food not by calories alone but by how much each food fills your stomach and satisfies you. By using the EMI, you'll learn how to eat as much as 200% more food than you now do—AND STILL LOSE WEIGHT!

Still skeptical? Consider that in the past 10 to 20 years we have decreased our caloric intake of food by approximately ten percent, yet obesity actually increased over the same period of time.(1,2) Consider also that Chinese people eat almost 30 percent more than Americans but weigh 20% less even after adjusting for height. (3) In fact, a stunning report out of Harvard University published in May, 1988 in the American Journal of Clinical Nutrition (4) states that in 8 out of 10 studies world-wide of the eating habits and weight of thousands, people who ate more actually weighed less, and only a part of that difference was attributable to exercise!

You can see, then, that a logical way to lose weight might well be to EAT MORE. In this book, you'll learn how to lose weight by eating all you want. You'll see how the latest scientific evidence suggests that in the long run you MUST eat more in order to weigh less!

This concept has been demonstrated in many experiences with my patients. One of them, Arthur H., was 6'1" and weighed 290 pounds when he first came to me for help. The first week on the Eat More Diet, Arthur lost 12 pounds—more than a pound a day! In the first three months Arthur lost 62 pounds, and he kept it off while eating more than he ever had in his life.

NO MORE YO-YO DIETING

What's even better is that because this is not a food deprivation diet, as are most other diets, there's less chance for yo-yo dieting. No more eating tiny portions of food or a stale powder for a period of time — losing weight — and then gorging yourself when the diet period is over — only to gain the weight back.

IF THEY CAN DO IT, YOU CAN DO IT TOO!

When I first saw Jane N., a 53-year-old secretary, she weighed 155 pounds. (She was only 5'1" tall and her normal weight was 105 pounds.) In six months, Jane lost 44 pounds—and she wasn't even trying to lose weight! What's even more remarkable is that it's been five years since she lost the weight, and she has kept the weight off.

A lot of people — including Jane, Arthur and other patients — have already demonstrated this. Another of my patients, Janice M. went on the program and lost 42 pounds in six months, and she was also on the diet for health reasons, not for weight loss! Kevin D. lost 53 pounds in four months. And for the first time in his life, he was on a diet that never left him hungry! IF THEY CAN DO IT, YOU CAN DO IT TOO!

THE POWER OF POSITIVE EATING

I emphasize the positive aspects of the Eat More Diet because it's important that you realize that you haven't picked up just another "quick fix" diet book. The trouble with diets is that you get "on" a diet, and eventually you'll get "off" one. Approximately 90 percent of all people regain every pound they've lost when they get "off" their diet. By contrast, the Eat More Diet is designed so that you can fully incorporate it into every aspect of your life and stay slim for good!

Earl M. started on the program in 1988. I closely monitored him for 30 days during which time he learned the principles of the Eat More Diet. At first, he was skeptical. "It's practically the opposite of what other doctors have told me," he said. But a few weeks into the program, he was saying, "I can't believe how simple it is—and it really works!" In that time, Earl lost 21 pounds. He learned how to choose and prepare foods, and learned to make certain he ate till he was completely full.

Earl continued the program on his own and 3 months later when he came in for another check-up, I was delighted to see that he had lost an additional 38 pounds. One year later he had lost 20 pounds more and was holding steady. He lost a whopping total of 79 pounds, and he's kept off every bit of it.

Jane N. proudly tells me, "My friends don't recognize me any more." Like the rest of my Eat More Diet patients, she has incorporated the Eat More Diet program into her life. At 49 years old, Jane was convinced she was going to be overweight forever. To make things even more difficult, she worked long hours at her government job, spent most of her work-time at a desk, and had trouble getting much exercise. "But I've not only lost 44 pounds on the Eat More Diet program," she now says, "I've gone from size 10 dresses to a size 4!" She also looks ten years younger than she did five years ago, when she first started on the program, and she hasn't gained back even one pound.

In the Eat More Diet program, we'll translate recent scientific studies to practical action as you discover how to achieve your ideal body weight while also maximizing your health. Since at least six of the ten leading causes of death are diet-related, you will also reap the added reward of decreasing your risks of many serious diseases. And—you're going to enjoy eating as much as you want while doing all this!

Startling, isn't it? And perhaps hard to accept, after a lifetime of listening to the propaganda that you have to deprive yourself in order to be slim. But—startling or not—this book will show you how to "eat yourself slim"!

CHAPTER 2

"The Sad Truth About Dieting In America"

THE SAD TRUTH IS—ALL DIETS WORK, AND ALL DIETS FAIL!

Let me assure you, you're not alone in your desire to be slim. At any given time in these United States, some 43 million people are on a diet to lose weight. (2)

Dieting in these United States was a $33 billion a year industry in 1990 (3) and probably approaches $50 billion in 1993. Most of these diets focus on the "quick fix" method of weight loss. Supermarket tabloids assure us that aliens have machines that can disintegrate fat with light rays, or that our favorite TV shows will help us lose weight—or that we can "easily" lose 32 pounds in nine days! Other more credible diets promise us the opulence and elegance of Beverly Hills, or the heady indulgence of champagne, or a diet that will change every facet of our lives in two or four or six or eight short days. Diet pills and liquid diets have been with us for decades now, with mixed and often alarming results.

In a 1986 article in Time Magazine, it was noted that over 90-percent of all Americans think they weigh too much. A large, well designed study done in 1990 called the "National Health Interview Survey" estimated that in the U.S., a staggering 28,688,881 or 40.1% of women were trying to lose weight and 15,009,011 or 23.3% of the men were trying to lose weight. (1)

But why then, in a country so preoccupied with weight loss, are so many people overweight?

One major reason is that almost all "diets" work, yet ultimately they fail. They produce gratifying weight loss but in the end, people gain it back. This holds for just about all diets, including the liquid diets such as the powdered formula diets, the liquid protein diets, low calorie diets, modified fasts, and drugs.

ONE REASON DIETS FAIL:
PEOPLE ARE FORCED TO EAT TOO LITTLE

The most common type of diet is a simple calorie restriction diet. To be sure, this type of diet works. However, one of the most common reasons these diets fail is that they fight your hunger by limiting calories or by "portion control," or focusing on a strictly limited amount of a single formula (e.g. powdered shake) or food (e.g. grapefruit diet) without taking into account your hunger or your body's metabolism.

If the calorie count is too low, your body fights back by changing its metabolic setpoint, that gauge which determines your metabolic activity and therefore the rate at which you burn calories. Your body thinks it is starving and slows itself down so that it can hold on to the calories you do eat. (4) In other words the hungrier you are, the more your body resists losing weight. In addition, many diets have you count calories without considering that most people will find it impractical to count calories for the rest of their lives. In my practice, just about every one of my patients who has tried to lose weight using this approach has been unable to continue it. Thus, counting calories becomes a short-term solution. These approaches are responsible, in part, for the "yo-yo effect" in which people diet and gain back weight repeatedly. (5)

ANOTHER PROBLEM: IS THE DIET HEALTHY?

Another type of diet is the diet that focuses on a single food (or food substitute). The diets in which some or all of the foods are replaced by a powdered shake, whether physician supervised or over-the-counter, fall into this category. These diets work to some extent either because they are easy to follow and strictly regimented, or they become so monotonous that the dieter deliberately forgets to eat and thus calories are automatically restricted. There are two problems with this type of diet:

first is the "yo-yo" effect that we've already mentioned; second, without eating a variety of real food, no one can stay on these diets and remain healthy for any significant period of time.

One of the best known types of diets is the low-carbohydrate diet or the "military diet." The unfortunate misconception that carbohydrates are fattening probably began with this type of diet. Some examples of the "military diet" include the Atkins diet and a variety of the Stillman diet. There are many others. In these diets, the basis for weight loss is "ketosis," which is a state in which the body burns fat because it is starving for carbohydrates. In other words, we lose weight because we are literally starving the body of necessary nutrients. As I said earlier, these diets work over the short term—but in an unhealthful way! (6) Furthermore, most of the foods on these diets are high in fat and cholesterol and therefore increase your risks of cardiovascular disease and cancer. Not a very good trade-off in return for the loss of a few pounds that will pile right back on as soon as you stop the diet. In addition, the high protein load taxes the kidneys and washes calcium out of the body, which among other things can promote osteoporosis.

There is no "quick fix" in dieting. Indeed, many variables play a part in every facet of our existence, and our weight is no exception. Some of the various factors involved are heredity, food intake, amount of exercise, your personal psychology, and your social support system. Social customs that dictate that most social gatherings revolve, somehow, around the ingestion of either food or alcohol is part of the problem. In fact, our social fixations with food might actually seem pathological, if viewed through the eyes of the proverbial Martian. The media, with all its tantalizing advertisements for food, is another part of the problem. TV food ads sensualize food, deify it, romanticize it—and generally reinforce our fixations. Something is seriously wrong with our relationships with the foods we eat when the foods we choose are what's killing us!

FOODS THAT HELP YOU LOSE WEIGHT

In this book, you'll learn which foods help you lose weight—fit foods—and which help you gain weight—fat foods. And this isn't an arbitrary labeling. You can identify these foods with the help of a simple tool that I developed, the "Eat More Index" (EMI). In addition, the diet I am about to share with you is based on the simplest logic and the support of scientific studies and the experience of populations around the world. But I'm not going to drag you through a library of research material, interesting though it might be. The simple purpose of this book is to show you how the summarized principles of all our human experience can help you lose weight—your excess weight—automatically.

Putting it as simply as possible, I intend to show you how to make your unwanted fat disappear, almost effortlessly! But in order to do this, let's start with understanding a few things about diets, and why they do and don't work.

CALORIES ARE **NOT** EQUAL

The main concept behind any conventional weight-loss program is:

Input minus output = weight loss (or gain)

That is, the number of calories you eat minus the number of calories you burn each day determines how much weight you gain or lose. I just want to remind you of the concept, because almost everyone who talks about or writes about weight loss uses this concept. Said another way, in order to lose weight, you have to eat fewer calories than you burn, or burn more calories than you eat. (Calories, by the way, are simply units of energy).

This 'input-output' concept is why most reputable weight loss programs ask you to count calories and limit portion size. And we've all become so familiar with this concept that we think it's a rock-solid principle, right?

WRONG! Recent research is changing our understanding about calories and finding that calories are not always equal. (7,8) It is providing us with the basis for an alternative to the tediousness of counting calories and trying to survive on gnat-like portions of food. The Eat More Diet takes these concepts and makes it practical for you to incorporate them into your daily life.

WHAT'S WRONG WITH CONVENTIONAL DIETS

There are four problems with most conventional approaches to weight loss which cause them to fail. First, they do not consider how to satisfy your hunger drive—they only aggravate it. Second, they do not take into account the whole food—the nutritional qualities, the type, the other components—but only consider the caloric content. Thirdly, they do not take into account your metabolic setpoint (a concept which will be covered in a later chapter, and which is vital to your weight gain or loss). Fourth, they presume that all calories are the same, regardless of what foods they come from, when surprising as it may seem, there is an big difference between them.

As you read further, you'll learn how to deal with these problems in an easy-to-follow program. You will learn how to melt your fat away by consuming food that satisfies your hunger while at the same time automatically decreasing the intake of calories— without counting them! You'll learn how to increase the output of calories WITH OR WITHOUT EXERCISE, while you are at the same time satisfying your hunger rather than depriving yourself of food. It will also teach you how to play an incredible trick on the arithmetic of calorie counting, so that most of your calories don't count toward making you fat!

So—get ready! Nice surprises lie ahead. The next three chapters explain the three main underlying concepts of the Eat More Diet and why they work. The chapters that follow show you exactly how to incorporate these principles into your life. Very soon you're going to learn how to EAT MORE AND WEIGH LESS, and at this very moment you're on your way to new health, new vitality, and a slimmer, trimmer you! So— LET'S GET STARTED!

CHAPTER 3

To Lose Weight,
FILL YOUR STOMACH!

HUNGER: FRIEND OR FOE?

What's the first thing you do when you're hungry? You grab a snack if you can. Or, if you can't, you probably spend some time thinking about food, fantasizing about it, anticipating the pleasure of soon indulging. Then you go about planning when and where you're going to eat.

In fact, the hunger drive is one of the most powerful drives in nature. It is central to the behavior of all living creatures, and if you think about it with regard to such beasts as lions and tigers, you know it's not something you can easily manipulate. One minute the big cat is your sleekest friend, the next—you're its lunch! The hunger drive is powerful. In fact, hunger is so powerful that it can even drive human beings to eat each other! So let's not try to fight it. Let's make it work for us.

Most diets do little or nothing to help us stop overeating because they try to fight the natural hunger drive. This is why just about all other weight loss diets require so much willpower. With the Eat More Diet, you need much less willpower because instead of fighting the extremely powerful hunger drive, you are allowed—even encouraged—to eat until you're satisfied!

COUNTING CALORIES? NONSENSE!

I know you've already breathed a sigh of relief that I haven't insisted you start counting calories. While we know that counting calories can work, we also know that it means a life-time of tedious calculations if our weight is to be maintained. It's a terrible and unnecessary price to pay. So we're not going to bother with this bit of nonsense, because almost nobody is going to keep counting calories for years and certainly not for the rest of their life. Remember, it's not enough to lose the weight, you must keep the weight off if you're really going to reach your goal of maximum health and perfect weight.

But if we don't count calories, what do we do?

TURN A NEGATIVE INTO A POSITIVE

As I said before, let's use our hunger to help us lose weight.

Consider this: There are three main biological drives that cause both people and animals to ingest the nutrients necessary to sustain life: breathing, thirst, hunger.

Now let me ask you: When was the last time you knew anyone who had a problem with breathing too much air? How about drinking too much water? Does your neighbor phone you and chat for hours about how she just can't seem to keep from breathing too much air or drinking too much water? "Help me, Betty, I'm drowning! I just pigged out on tap-water!" It doesn't happen, does it?

So—at least we don't have to concern ourselves with over-breathing and over-watering. Why, then, do we have an entire culture obsessed with and plagued by over-eating? Were we designed with our thirst drives and breathing apparatus with no mistakes, yet somehow with a major defect when it came to hunger? Not likely. We have survived over millennia with no such problem and the mortar and bricks and other matter with which we rebuild our bodies are put in place through breathing, drinking and eating—in other words, what you eat today is what you'll be tomorrow! And it is what you choose to eat and drink that can determine whether that's good news or bad news.

THE SCIENCE OF HUNGER

The science of human hunger and appetite can be extremely complex. Thousands of experiments have been done on nearly every aspect of these intertwining subjects. (I'm sure you can imagine why). But here I'll try to simplify hunger and appetite into two main mechanisms. The first main mechanism of hunger satisfaction is nerve impulses to the appetite center of the brain, and the second main mechanism is substances carried in the blood stream to this center. Nerve impulses to the brain come from the smell, and taste of food and the sensation of chewing, swallowing and filling of the stomach with food. The blood stream carries substances that satisfy hunger such as hormones and food substances such as carbohydrate, fat and protein. (1)

The hunger or appetite center is found in an area of your brain known as the hypothalamus. This is your central satiety system (satiety is another word for hunger satisfaction) which tells you when to eat and when to stop eating. The following list shows the mechanisms that send messages to the central satiety system and satisfy our hunger. They are:

I. NERVE IMPULSES

    A.   Sensory Quality of Food

        1.   Taste/Smell/Appearance
        2.   Texture/Chewing
        3.   Swallowing

    B.   Fullness of the stomach
        (due to mass of food eaten)

II. SUBSTANCES IN THE BLOOD STREAM

    A.   Stomach hormones
        (due to fullness of the stomach)

        1.   Bombesin
        2.   Cholecystokinin

        3.   Somatostatin
        4.   Gastro-intestinal Peptide (GIP)

  B.   Nutrients

        1.   Glucose
        2.   Amino Acids
        3.   Purines
        4.   Fatty Acids

  C.   Hormonal signals from other organs

        1.   Liver
        2.   Fat tissue
        3.   Glands

Unless you've just eaten, when you see, smell and taste food you get hungry. But as you continue to smell and taste the food, your hunger begins to dissolve and your appetite is gradually satisfied—at least for the moment. The acts of chewing and swallowing are a part of the process, and they also contribute to your satisfaction.

As food reaches your stomach, it begins to fill it up. The degree to which it will be filled depends primarily upon the volume and mass of the food itself. As the stomach stretches, it sends a signal up the vagus nerve to the brain's hunger center: "Stomach filling up, you can relax. This body won't starve just yet." But this is only a part of the complex process of hunger satiation. A stretched or stretching stomach also seems to secrete a hormone known as 'bombesin,' which also sends a chemical message to the brain: "Satisfied here, you can quit eating!" (Surgeons who perform stomach stapling operations or insert balloons in stomachs to cure obesity rely on this mechanism.)

The absorption of nutrients also satisfies hunger. Blood sugar, amino acids, and purines all tell the brain that there is food coming in and, therefore, it need not send out hunger signals to the body at the moment. These nutrients and others we may not be aware of also trigger the stomach wall's production of cholecystokinin and somatostatin, which is what actually stimulates the vagus nerve to tell the brain that it is no longer hungry.

TWO MAIN FACTORS IN FOOD THAT SATISFY HUNGER

For the purpose of selecting foods to help you lose weight, we can distill the effect of food on this complex mechanism of satisfying hunger down to two main factors.

1. FOOD MASS, OR VOLUME. Eating a large volume of food requires a lot of chewing, tasting and swallowing; this already starts to make you satisfied. It also causes the stomach to stretch and signals the brain via the vagus nerve and stomach hormones that it is satisfied. In addition, eating more tends to take more time. This allows the many other satiety mechanisms the time they need to work on the brain, so it will in turn signal you to feel full before you eat more than you can handle.

2. NUTRIENTS. Eating the right amount and mix of nutrients satisfies hunger and also triggers hormones and other organs to signal the brain that it is satisfied and to stop the eating behavior.

Most diets ignore these factors. They totally ignore Factor #1, and the body's need for food volume, and they put you in the almost impossible position of doing battle against your own hunger drive in order to lose weight. It's a battle most people can't win. They also uniformly focus on counting calories and assume all calories are the same, thus ignoring Factor #2.

The Eat More Diet program utilizes both Factor #1 by showing you how to fill your stomach and satisfy your hunger as well as Factor #2 by showing you what to eat that will make the calories you eat satisfy you, contribute as little as possible to weight gain and make you lose weight automatically.

IF YOU'RE OVERWEIGHT, MOST LIKELY IT'S NOT BECAUSE YOU EAT TOO MUCH

What most diet experts would have you believe isn't altogether true. They would have you believe that overweight is caused by overeating. This may be so in a few individuals who have true eating disorders; however, some very good studies suggest that most of us who are overweight eat too little! When I say

FOOD CHANGES OVER TIME
Fat and sugar consumption have increased at the expense of complex carbohydrates

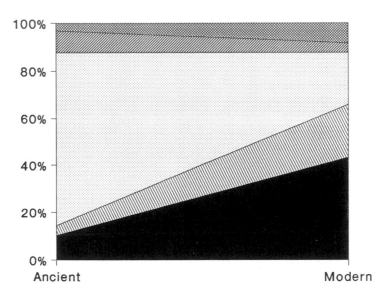

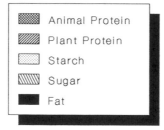

Modern estimates based on U.S. 1980
Welsh SO, J Am Dietetic Assn 1982;81:120

too little, I mean too little in terms of ounces or pounds of food and the volume it occupies in our stomachs.

Let's look at it this way. We developed to our present form, with a breathing mechanism, a thirst mechanism, and a hunger mechanism, and these were based upon what the air, water, and food was like during that process of development. The hunger, breathing, and food mechanisms in the human body haven't changed in the one million or so years during which humanity has been a separate species. Neither has the air and water changed substantially, despite modern pollution. But—during the past 100 to 200 years—our food has radically changed!

Just since 1900, the consumption in the U.S. of what as been the staple foods of humanity has decreased dramatically. Wheat consumption is down by 41%, fresh vegetable consumption is down by 23% and corn consumption is down by 84%. We have replaced it with high-fat and thus low bulk foods. For example, beef consumption is up by 44%, fat and oil consumption up by 49%, poultry up by 344% and cheese consumption up by 440%! (2)

OUR ANCESTORS WEREN'T FAT

There are no indications that our ancestors were fat, despite the fact that they ate a lot of food. Our ancestors ate whole foods, primarily grains and vegetables, and occasionally hard-won fish and animal food. For thousands upon thousands of years, they ate this way.

Our bodies were designed to eat the "ancient" food—mostly unprocessed grains and vegetables. Our whole dietary systems, from our teeth to our stomach size to the length of our intestines—even to our very brains—were (and are still) designed to function best with these kinds of foods. Meat eaters, such as tigers and lions, have short intestines and strong, sharp canine teeth. You and I have long intestines— like all other herbivores and omnivores. We have 28 veg- etable-and-grain-crushing teeth, but only 4 meat-eating teeth. From the very structure of our bodies, it's apparent that we are designed to eat primarily plant-type foods and very small amounts of animal flesh.

WHAT WENT WRONG

But within the past hundred or so years, a dietary revolution occurred along with the industrial revolution, and our bodies didn't have time to adapt. Now, we're using the wrong foods. Deadly foods. Foods that are destroying the machine they are intended to energize. Without realizing it, we've gone through a dietary revolution, and the wrong side won! We've changed from eating whole grains, vegetables, and occasional wild game to canned goods, and refined foods. Furthermore, modern foods have been processed or chemicalized until there's not much actual 'food' left in the substances we put into our mouths.

An event that seemed to be a blessing for mankind has proved to be a nutritional disaster. We tried to extend the shelf life of food and reduce spoilage and food hazards such as botulism. While we succeeded to some extent in making food safer from the standpoint of infectious disease, we have not made food safer from an overall perspective. Instead, we have created an eating pattern that contributes to nearly 70% of all the deaths in America. Put simply, when it came to our food, we outsmarted ourselves by inventing machines and other technology which changed the character and the quality of the foods we need to survive. As a result, we don't eat enough to satisfy our hunger drive in a natural way and we are killing ourselves in the process.

PROGRESS IS KILLING US

With the advent of our wonderful machines and their marvelous abilities, we began to tamper with our food. We started making our foods easier to preserve, easier to cook, easier on the eyes, and more pleasing to the palate—or so we believed. Today we have refrigerators which allow us to eat high fat meats, poultry and fish at every meal as our main dish. We even grade the highest fat cuts of meat as the highest grade. Eating such animal foods causes us to eat a small amount of food for a large amount of calories. And unfortunately, we have encouraged the consumption of foods that are high in fat and cholesterol that contribute to the leading causes of death in America.

In addition, we suddenly had refined, canned, packaged foods laden with artificial chemicals, flavorings, and colorings. While our ancestors ate whole foods such as whole-wheat breads, brown rice and whole vegetables, we eat white bread with all the nutrients milled out, white rice which is equally depleted of nutrients, and refined sugars which we nutritionists call "empty calories." No longer do we get the vitamins, minerals, fiber, and micro-nutrients that help us function optimally and combat disease. We now peel, refine, mill, chemicalize and package our foods, and most of us have little regard for any component of those foods save for convenience and taste. We also use a smaller part of any particular food than we would have before this deadly trend began. There are thousands of such foods.

In fact, American food is now so processed that practically no food is real anymore. Most members of the food industry are concerned only about what looks and tastes best so that the largest number of people will buy it. What's healthy is rarely a major consideration. Sometimes manufacturers put the caloric content on the packaging, in order to placate more weight-conscious customers, and sometimes—after much social pressure—they even disclose the fat and salt contents. But what they don't tell you is that half of the food we think we're purchasing is actually missing! A large part of the food we need to satisfy our hunger has been processed out, left on the factory floor, burnt up into thin air, or otherwise tampered with. As a result, too many of us eat more unhealthy food and are literally eating ourselves to death.

To better explain this, let's look at an example, fat (or oil, which is nothing more than liquid fat). We all know that meats and poultry have a lot of fat—today—that is. For example, an average steak is 60% to 70% fat calories depending on the cut. This is assuming domesticated beef that is sedentary and fed cattle feed. In ancient times, human beings ate meat that was as low as 14% fat calories. This is because the wild game they ate fed in the wild and was active and had a lot of exercise. When you eat a fatty steak, you are eating about 62% less food for the same number of calories as you do when you eat piece of wild game. This is because fat has so many calories for such little food.

A THOUSAND EARS OF FAT

Even vegetable sources of food can be fatty, too, if processed or fried. Vegetable oils are the most extreme example as they are 100% fat and in a sense are the most highly processed of foods. In order to make one day's calories worth of corn oil or 2,500 calories, 9.7 oz or .6 pounds, at least 377 ears of corn have to be processed assuming 75% efficiency. If you want to make a quart of oil, it takes 1,185 ears.

Today, everything from the hamburger at your local restaurant to Mother's home-made French fries are cooked in vegetable oils. Instead of getting the 1,185 ears of corn into our stomachs, to process slowly and get the full nutritional value from, we get the oil. Our bodies were not designed to ingest and digest this much vegetable oil. This simple fact proves itself by causing many human diseases, one of which we call 'obesity'!

Eating oil also interferes with standard dieting because it is so little food. It causes that horrible hollow feeling you get when you start cutting down on food volume. It will drive you to the nearest chocolate bar, hamburger stand, or refrigerator. The way to keep your hands out of the potato chips is to have a full stomach, which in turn satiates your hunger drive! The EMI helps you do just that.

EATING 200% MORE FOOD WITH LESS CALORIES

Just think about the photograph you see on the opposite page which compares the hamburger and fries with the plate of Eat More Diet food. Are these two meals equivalent? Of course not. Which one will fill you up faster? There's no question about it, is there? And—which one will leave your stomach partly empty? Which will leave your body starving for something more to eat? No doubt about that, either, is there?

Think about the photograph again. The cheeseburger, fries, and shake (bottom picture) has 1,195 calories. The Eat More Diet food (top picture) has 1,125 calories. Yet the burger meal weighs only 636 grams, while the Eat More Diet meal weighs a full 1,885 grams — almost three times more food by weight!

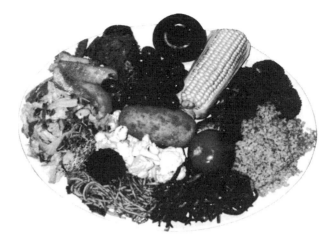

1,125 Calories
1,883 Grams

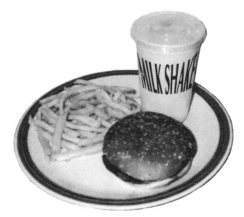

1,195 Calories
636 Grams

Nutrition aside, we are nevertheless actually starving for more bulk in our stomach when we eat the burger, whereas with the Eat More Diet meal, you get everything you need, including good nutrition. Only when we see real food next to the fake food do we begin to see what's happening.

FILLING YOUR STOMACH WITHOUT CALORIES

A major characteristic of the foods our ancestors ate is that they were high in bulk and low in fat. They contain large amounts of fiber and water, neither of which have any calories, but both of which nevertheless have the ability to make you feel full. In addition, the overall fat content of these foods was about 10 to 15 percent fat. By contrast, the foods we eat today are just that—fat! Today, the composition of our diet is approximately 38 to 40 percent fat! And to compound the culinary crime, we also eat volumes of refined white flour and white sugar, which are devoid of most of the nutrients and bulk we need to make us feel full and satisfied.

Because of fast food, processed food and tampered-with food, we are missing out on much of the fiber, vitamins, minerals and trace elements that we desperately need. And a large part of our health—or lack thereof—shows up as obesity. As I said before, and it can't be stressed too strongly, that obesity is a signal from nature that something's wrong with your diet. Strange as it may sound, an obese person is starving for the bulk and nutrients that have been taken out of our foods. We overeat because we eat too little! Our bodies need foods that are far different in composition and texture from what we eat today. Our stomachs are constantly crying out for enough food to fill us up at every single meal. If you choose foods that are devoid of natural bulk and nutrition, you can expect to be unhealthy and overweight. However, if you fill up with the right foods, you can eat as much or more than you do now, and you can expect better health and a slimmer you. In other words, starting now, you can EAT MORE AND WEIGH LESS!

PUTTING THIS APPROACH TO THE TEST

Research that we conducted in 1989 in Hawaii confirmed this paradoxical approach that I had been using in my private prac-

tice that we believed was supported by medical literature —
that is, automatic weight loss while eating more food. In this
study, we hypothesized that if the right foods were selected,
individuals would wind up eating more food but losing weight.
Twenty native Hawaiian men and women who were obese were
placed on a non-calorie restricted diet made up of foods which
were high in EMI. They were allowed to eat until they were
satisfied. In just three weeks while eating as much as they
wanted, they lost an average of 17.1 pounds, and they did it
without counting calories and eating as much as they wanted.
What was even more significant is that, just as we predicted,
they were eating MORE FOOD, about 4.1 pounds of food per
day! (3)

Another team of researchers did a similar study in 1981 in
which they placed people into two groups. One group ate the
high-fat Standard American Diet (SAD, which was about 42
percent fat at that time), while the other ate what they called
the "low energy density diet" (LED diet). The LED diet was
low in fat and high in fiber so that the caloric density was very
low. In fact, this diet was 15 percent fat, which is similar to
the percentage of fat found in the diets of our previous generations.

The experimenters not only counted the calories that each
group consumed, they also recorded their satiety—the amount
of satisfaction and fullness they experienced. They found that
the SAD group (42 percent fat) had to consume about 3,000
calories per day to keep satisfied. But to the LED diet group
ate only about 1,570 calories per day with essentially the same
level of satisfaction and fullness! And as in our study, none of
those in the study counted calories, and they all ate as much as
they wanted. (4,5,6)

The difference occurred because the people in the LED group
were eating foods that were bulkier and which their own bodies
were designed to eat! When this is done, hunger mechanisms
work properly, and thereby regulate the number of calories that
we eat automatically. And happily, we don't feel hungry while
this is happening, nor do we feel deprived. We simply lose
weight naturally, until we've reached our ideal body weight.
Incredible, isn't it? Nevertheless, this is precisely the way it works.

What's even more astonishing is this: if you weighed the food the two groups ate, you'd find that the group eating less calories (1,570 calories compared to 3,000 calories) was actually eating more food in terms of weight (4.1 pounds vs. 2.76 pounds), while maintaining the same level of satisfaction. (Remember the quarter pound burger!) In other words, they were eating more and weighing less.

THE PROOF IS IN OUR DAILY BREAD

In England, another experiment demonstrated this using a single type of food: bread. Two groups of people were given bread to eat. Both groups were told to eat as much as they wanted till they were full. The only difference between the two groups was that one group was given whole wheat bread (which contains lots of fiber), while the other was given white bread (which is a more processed food, and contains little fiber). Guess which group ate more calories? Right! The whole wheat group ate fewer calories than the white bread group, even though both groups were equally satisfied with regard to appetite! (7)

The logical reason for this is that there was more fiber in the whole wheat bread, which made the people feel more satisfied with fewer calories because their stomachs were full. A similar study was done comparing apples, apple sauce and apple juice and they found that the whole apple with undisturbed fiber satisfied the most. (8) Also, fiber helps slow absorption of food, which in turn decreases the amount of the hormone, insulin, that your body requires in response to blood sugar. This in turn decreases the production of fat. This slow absorption also means that the body feels satisfied for longer periods of time so that the craving to snack is minimized.

FILLING UP ON FIBER

What is fiber? It's the undigestible part of plant-type foods such as fruit, grains, and vegetables. Because it is non-digestible, it provides no calories and stays in your stomach and intestines, making you feel full and satisfied. Eventually, fiber gets eliminated without being absorbed. This is one major reason why eating whole foods helps you eat more and weigh less. Fiber absorbs water and provides bulk in your stomach and intestines. It makes you feel full faster because of this bulk, and works on your natural mechanism of feeling satisfied.

Besides promoting weight loss, studies have shown that fiber has many beneficial effects on human health. For example, cancer of the colon is found in smaller numbers in societies which have a high fiber diet. Fiber also helps form bulk in the stool. Having bulk in the stool helps food move through the digestive tract with ease. This helps eliminate constipation and hemorrhoids. It prevents straining at the stool and thus decreases the incidence of diverticular disease. It also decreases the possibility of blocking the appendix and thus prevents appendicitis. Other studies have shown that fiber helps lower cholesterol and sex hormone levels levels by decreasing absorption and increasing elimination of these substances in the stool. This should help decrease the risk of heart attacks, premenstrual syndrome, and other health hazards.

In other words, you want to be able to lose weight while at the same time have a full stomach. You need to eat foods that will fill you up without filling you out. Just as our ancestors ate foods that were composed almost totally of whole foods and thus were high in bulk, we must learn to do the same, so that we may maintain our most healthy weights and eliminate the diet-related diseases that are plaguing our country.

FORGET COUNTING CALORIES!

So—stick to the Eat More Diet and forget—forever—about counting calories. You can use the EMI or "Eat More Index" of Food to help you select foods that are high in volume and nutrition and low in calorie density! You'll get more high-octane fuel and satisfaction per calorie if you give up the refined foods—the fat foods—and return to the fit foods of our ancestors. So, to lose weight, simply fill your stomach. But use high EMI foods so that they help you lose weight.

CHAPTER 4

The One Category of Food to Avoid to Lose Weight For Good!

This is it. The one category of food you have to avoid if you want to lose weight for good without being hungry.

From all I've said earlier, you must have already guessed what is the dietary villain causing much of the health and obesity problems. But I can't emphasize this point too much. To lose weight, you don't have to count calories, you don't have to eat small portions of food and remain hungry all the time. All you have to do is realize that there's one main reason why people in these United States are becoming more and more obese while at the same eating less and less food! That reason is—FAT! Not the kind of fat you carry on your body, but the kind you shove into your mouth!

Fats and oils both fall into the category of dietary fat. These are the culprits. As I pointed out above, we're eating more and more fats these days than ever before, and we're also getting fatter and fatter. Not to mention sicker and sicker. To belabor the point—you really are what you eat! Eat fat and you're going to be fat. It's just that simple.

FAT FAILS TO FILL YOU, SO IT SATISFIES YOU THE LEAST!

Many health professionals say that fat is the most satisfying food. This is a misleading statement however, because they are thinking ounce for ounce fat is indeed more satisfying than many other foods. This is because there are so many calories in fat. However, from the standpoint of weight loss, we must look at satisfaction per calorie, not satisfaction per gram of food. Let's look at the logic as to why fat is the least satisfying of all.

Fat has 9 calories per gram. In fact, recent studies suggest that it may even be closer to 10 calories per gram. (1) When we compare it to starches in their whole form, which are approximately 0.6 to 1 calorie per gram, you can see that it doesn't take much fat or oil to quickly exceed the amount of calories that we need to eat each day. (Note that refined carbohydrates such as white flour and sugar are about 4 calories per gram) A little simple arithmetic tells us that we can, indeed, eat nine to ten times more whole starch than fat, and end up with the same amount of calories! And you're actually better off eating ten times more complex carbohydrate because such calories actually count less that fat calories in terms of causing you to be fat. In any case you should eat more whole complex carbohydrate foods if for no other reason than that fats are hard on your health as well as your scales.

Fat also has the dubious distinction of having the lowest "Eat More Index" (EMI) value of any food. I'll explain the EMI fully in a later chapter, but let me give you a preview of this index which I devised to help you examine which foods satisfy you the most per calorie. The EMI number is generally the number of pounds of food it takes to provide 2,500 calories or one day's worth of calories for an average active woman or average inactive man. Thus, the higher the EMI number of a food, that is, the more pounds of food it takes to provide your daily calories, the more likely you are to be satisfied by eating a selected food. Fat has an EMI value of 0.61—the lowest EMI value of any food. In other words it takes 0.61 pounds (9.7 ounces) of this food—the smallest amount as compared to any other food to provide an average day's 2,500 calories. Thus, it satisfies you the least per calorie.

SO—WHAT IS FAT AND WHY DOES IT WORK THAT WAY?

Fat is actually a means by which people, animals and plants store their reserve energy. It is an oily substance which is not water soluble. It is also highly concentrated in energy so we can keep a great deal of energy stored in a relatively light material. This is why such a small amount of fat contains so many calories. Since fats are the storage forms of reserve energy for plants and animals, it makes sense that they contain the highest amounts of calories per gram.

Plants store their energy in ways similar to humans and animals, except that plants have a much higher concentration of polyunsaturated fats. At room temperature, these fatty substances become liquid, so we call them oils. We eat many types of these oils: soy-bean oil, cottonseed oil, sesame oil, and so forth. By contrast, animal fats are solid at room temperature. This is because animal fats are high in saturated fats. While saturated fats are worse for you in terms of raising cholesterol and your risk of heart disease, don't forget that both are equal in terms of calories.

FAT TURNS INTO FAT

Aside from the fact that fat has more calories per gram than any other food, there's an additional reason not to eat fat. Recent studies indicate that dietary fat turns into body fat far more easily than do any other nutrients. As you've already seen, your body uses only 3% of the calories from dietary fats to convert them to body fat, whereas it uses 23% of the starches' calories to do the same thing. Again—YOU ARE WHAT YOU EAT! The more fat you eat, the fatter you'll be. IT'S JUST THAT SIMPLE!

This conclusion is reinforced by certain experiments with mice. In 1985, researchers placed different populations of mice on diets that differed with regard to percentages of fat. One group ate a diet that was 15% fat, a second group ate a diet that was 35% fat, and a third a diet that was 45% fat. All these mice were allowed to eat as much as they wanted during the experiment. (2)

The researchers found that the 15% fat group had only a 3% incidence of obesity, whereas the 35% fat group had a 26% incidence of obesity, and the 45% fat group had a 48% incidence of obesity! This means that populations of mice who were allowed to eat as much as they wanted became obese in direct relation to the amount of fat in their diet! It seems that in mice, the amount of fat in the diet determines the amount of fat on the body.

The same relationship between dietary fat and body fat appears to hold true for people. Dr. Dennis Burkitt of Oxford University noted that in Africa, Australia, and Micronesia—in virtually every country in the world that's seen a rise in dietary fat intake as a result of change in dietary habit—the rise of obesity occurs in direct proportion to the amount of dietary fat these populations begin to eat. (3) It's as if the amount of fat in the diet seems to alter and determine the set-point for each individual. In other words, the amount of fat in a culture's diet seems to determine the amount of individual obesity—with regard to entire populations of people! (4,5,6)

Said more precisely, THE MORE FAT YOU CONSUME, THE MORE FAT YOU'LL RETAIN ON YOUR BODY. Back to the old-but-accurate cliche: YOU ARE WHAT YOU EAT!

More recently, studies on humans show that fats make you fat. A team of researchers at Harvard University conducted the largest study on diet and disease of its type in history. Ninety thousand women in the "Nurses' Health Study" were surveyed on diet and other factors. Their startling findings regarding weight loss and diet were that there was NO CORRELATION BETWEEN CALORIES AND OBESITY. (7) However, they did find a correlation between dietary fat and obesity.

Other human studies have shown that fats make people fat and other sources of calories, i.e., protein and carbohydrates don't. In 1988, a researcher named Acheson demonstrated what happens when you overfeed humans with carbohydrate. In this experiment, he monitored 12 individuals to demonstrate what happened when they were fed a regular mixed diet and then added up to 1,000 extra calories of carbohydrate per day to their food supply. The metabolic studies showed that the extra calories were burned off or turned into glycogen (which is easy to burn off) and ONLY 4% OF THE STARCH CALORIES TURNED INTO FAT. At the same time the body continued to burn fat and the result was a net decrease in body fat. (8,9) Another research team headed by J.P. Flatt demonstrated that when individuals are overfed dietary fat, the amount of fat burned stayed the same and at least 21% or about FIVE TIMES MORE calories turned into fat. (10)

This phenomenon could explain the puzzling finding that there was no correlation between calories and obesity among different populations in a well designed study. In fact one researcher concluded that:

> "... [C]alorie differences are not the major cause of the variations in obesity in these men.
> ...[T]otal fat, saturated fatty acids, and monounsaturated fatty acids were positively related with body fatness whereas total carbohydrate, fiber, and plant protein were negatively correlated" (11)

In the study that we conducted in Hawaii, weight loss was automatic with a diet that was 7% fat. (12) Similar results were obtained by others using a low-fat diets ranging up to 20% fat calories in their studies. (13,14,15).

It follows, then, that the less fat you eat, the less fat you become. Which doesn't mean you have to go without food, as these studies have shown. Thankfully, in the Eat More Diet, those wonderful high EMI foods easily fill your stomach.

So, if you stick mostly to high EMI foods, to high complex carbohydrate foods, and high fiber vegetables; and avoid fatty foods, you'll lose weight effortlessly, and without hunger. You won't have to worry about restricting your caloric intake, you won't have to study all those calorie tables and calculate formulas to figure out how many calories are in a food. EAT LESS FAT—AND YOU'LL ALMOST ALWAYS BE EATING RIGHT to lose weight.

THE MOST IMPORTANT FOOD FORMULA
• THE FAT FINDER FORMULA •

But how do we avoid excess fat when so much of it is hidden in the foods we eat? Here's a simple formula that can help to reveal hidden fat. I consider it to be the MOST IMPORTANT

FOOD FORMULA that I teach because it might save your life! I call it the FAT FINDER FORMULA. Why do we need a formula? A formula is needed because there is so much concealed fat in our food that it's time we learned how to find it so we can avoid it.

Part of the problem is in how fat is reported on labels. Most foods don't report fat in percent of fat calories. This is unfortunate because national goals and guidelines for fat intake are described by percent of fat calories. Most foods are reported in grams fat or percent of fat by weight. This leads to very misleading labeling of fat in foods. Not only is it misleading but it is dangerous because in the long run, too much fat kills millions of people.

EXAMPLES OF HIDDEN FAT

Two percent milk is a good example. Two percent milk sounds like it's "98% fat free." The truth is that 2% milk is actually 35% fat as a percent of calories. The advertisers never bothered to tell you that the 2% is calculated by weight and not by caloric value which is how it should be reported. They also don't tell you that whole milk is 3.3% fat by weight (55% by calories). Another good example is the famous "91% fat free" burger which is actually nearly 50% fat by calories. Other examples of hidden fats are 5% fat ham which is actually 39% fat by calories and chicken hot dogs which claim to be less that 20% fat but that are actually 68% fat by calories (better than beef franks that are 83% fat).

How do we find the fat in our foods? What I like to use is a formula which I call the "Fat Finder Formula". It's based on the simple fact that fats (both saturated and unsaturated) are 9 calories per gram. So the formula is as simple as this. Look at a food label and take the grams of fat and multiply by nine (grams fat x 9). Then divide this number by the total calories and the number you get is the proportion of fat in the diet.

Grams of fat x 9/total calories = proportion of fat calories; multiply by 100 and you get percent fat calories.

Remember that while national guidelines currently recommend a fat intake of less than 30% of calories, more and more experts agree that a safer level is around 10 to 15% in fat. Even those who promote 30% fat as a target concede that a lower level is more desirable and that the 30% fat target is a compromise because they believe that most of the general public will not accept a lower fat calorie percentage. Personally, I don't like to compromise when it comes to people's health.

Let me repeat:

The FAT FINDER FORMULA IS:

Grams fat x 9/total calories x 100 = percent fat calories

Let's take some examples.

2 percent milk has 4.7 gm of fat and 121 calories total.

Using the formula we get:

4.7 grams x 9 = 42.3 calories.
42.3 calories divided by 121 calories = .35

.35 x 100 = 35 percent fat calories.

Other examples:

Hot Dogs (per wiener):

16.8 grams fat x 9 = 151 (calories from fat)
divided by 183 total calories = .83
or 83 percent fat calories.

Let's see if chicken hot dogs are any better.

8.8 grams fat x 9 = 79 (calories from fat)
divided by 116 total calories = .68
or 68 percent fat calories.

Luncheon Meat (1 slice):

4 grams fat x 9 = 36 (calories from fat)
divided by 50 total calories = .72
         or 72 percent fat calories.

Sweet Potato:

.13 grams fat x 9 = 1.17 (calories from fat)
divided by 118 total calories = .01
         or 1 percent fat calories.

Now consider that the diet of millions of people of many cultures who are naturally slim is roughly 10 to 20 percent in fat content. Also consider that almost all whole, unprocessed food have fat contents at this level or even less.

If you can learn to use the Fat Finder Formula (or the fat portion of the EMI table) in your shopping and food selections, you might find how much fat there is in foods that you may have thought were "low fat." You might find yourself choosing foods different from what you choose now. You are also inadvertently lowering your cholesterol level and inadvertently lowering your risk of cancer. And perhaps best of all, if you keep your total fat intake from 10 to 20 percent of your calories, you may find yourself Eating More and still losing weight automatically.

HOW MUCH FAT CAN I EAT

The Eat More, Weigh Less™ Diet
FAT GRAM Approach

For people who have a difficult time watching the fat in their diet, it may be useful to use what I call the "Fat Gram" approach. This is one good way to help keep you on the Eat More Diet. In this approach, you count the grams of fat, not the calories that you eat. After all, fat is what makes you fat. The less fat in your food, the less fat on your body.

It's as simple as that. One of the best ways to lose weight using this concept is to limit your fat intake to approximately

10 percent of your calories. Now remember, I didn't say limit the amount of food, or limit the calories you eat—just the amount of fat. The way to do this is to estimate the amount of calories you will be eating in a day and multiply by .1. For example, if you are eating 2,000 calories a day, your fat intake should be 2,000 x .1 = 200 calories to make 10 percent. To translate this to grams of fat, divide by 9 and you get 22 grams. (Essentially, this is using the FFF in reverse). Here are some values calculated for various daily calorie intake levels and fat percentages.

Grams of fat in 10% fat and 15% fat diets

Total Daily Calories	10% fat diet	15% fat diet
1,500	17 gm fat	25 gm fat
2,000	22 gm fat	33 gm fat
2,500	28 gm fat	42 gm fat
3,000	33 gm fat	50 gm fat

The above table indicates the maximum amount of fat you can eat to make a 10 percent fat diet and a 15 percent fat diet depending on how many calories you eat per day. In general, for a ballpark estimate, women eat roughly 1,500 to 2,500 calories per day depending on activity and body size. Men eat roughly 2,000 to 3,000 calories per day depending on activity and body size. The more active you are, the larger your body size, the higher your daily calorie consumption.

Thus, no matter what you eat, if you limit your fat intake to 22 grams per day or less, if you are an average woman with average activity eating 2,000 calories or more, your fat intake will be 10 percent or less of your intake. This should help you to lose weight automatically. I caution you to still look at the EMI chart so that you don't wind up eating highly refined or high sugar content foods such as jelly beans which have no fat but are potentially fattening because of low EMI values of high sugar content foods.

Read labels carefully for the amount of fat they contain. Remember that staying on the Eat More Diet plan will result in a roughly 10 percent fat diet if you limit the oils in the cooking.

Why not start right now. NO MORE FAT FOODS! This is the one category of food you have to learn to avoid. And—if you can and do avoid them....

GET READY TO GET SLIM
AND STAY THAT WAY FOR GOOD!

CHAPTER 5

Lose Weight While You Sleep

In this chapter you'll learn one of the secrets of why people Eat More and still Weigh Less. At this point, the EAT MORE DIET program gets about as easy as anything could possibly be, because now I'm going to teach you how to lose weight while you're asleep! And no, I'm not going to suggest that you poison your body with fat blockers, or with any of the other "magic bullets" that people keep using to try to lose weight. I also promised to show you how to become healthier, remember? And one thing to remember about bullets, magic or otherwise, is that they are not natural and they can harm you.

Slumber, on the other hand, restores you, both physically and mentally. Furthermore, the principle I am going to share with you will also work when you're awake and just relaxing, such as right now while you're sitting down reading a book.

YOUR FAT FURNACE

How does this principle work? Your body is always burning energy, even when you're sleeping. This energy is in the form of calories, and they are burned at a certain rate. Scientists call the rate at which calories are burned while you're at rest your basal metabolic rate (BMR). We'll call this your "Fat Furnace", because it can burn your fat away.

Fortunately, there are simple, healthy ways in which you can increase the rate at which you burn that energy, even while you sleep! You don't have to be thinking about what you're doing, or worrying about it. If you make a few preliminary adjustments, it will work by itself, burning off calories automatically!

There are three main things that you can control to do this: 1. how much you eat, 2. what you eat, 3. how much you play. We'll go through them one by one. But first, let's talk about the fat furnace. The scientific explanation of how we can automatically burn calories is actually quite simple. Scientists have identified four major factors which determine how much weight we lose while we sleep (or at any other time except during exercise). These factors control the setting of our Fat Furnace by determining the rate at which our bodies burn energy, including fat energy. One of these factors can't be changed, but the other three are amazingly simple to use in order to help you lose weight—even while you sleep!

The unchangeable factor which determines how much fat your fat furnace burns is your hereditary metabolic rate. (1,2) This rate is genetically determined, and try though we might, we'll never change it. Everyone has a different genetic BMR, and—just as you might have suspected—this gives some people the edge when it comes to weight control. This is why some people never seem to gain weight, no matter what they eat, while others seem to eat very little and are nevertheless obese. But—though we can't change it, we can overcome its effect to a large degree by the way we eat. While "overweight runs in my family" is a great excuse, there is so much we can do to be slim in spite of familial tendency.

One of the best ways we can compensate for a tendency to be overweight is by using three weight-loss factors to their maximal extent to help you lose weight even in your sleep. Let's go through them, one by one.

1. HOW MUCH YOU EAT: This is the first way you can reset your fat furnace. Eating enough makes use of a mechanism known as "adaptive thermogenesis." Basically, it is the body's way of adapting to the conditions around it: lack of food, changes in climate, changes in diet. "Thermogenesis" means the generation of heat or the burning of calories. Adaptive thermogenesis is partly responsible for people regaining a lot of weight after dieting, and is also known as the "Yo-Yo Effect," wherein people keep dieting and gaining, dieting and gaining, time after time. It works thus: If the hunger center in the brain senses that it is short of food (such as in starvation

states or dieting), it will cause the Fat Furnace to burn more slowly so that the body will burn its energy—fat—more slowly, thus precluding starvation. This adaptation in our Fat Furnace is probably nature's way of helping us to stay alive during starvation, extreme temperatures and other prevailing conditions. Step #1 in this chapter shows you how to make "adaptive thermogenesis" work for you instead of against you.

STEP #1: EAT ENOUGH: Make adaptive thermogenesis work for you. Your basal metabolic rate can change in response to the way you eat. Thus, it is important to satisfy your hunger so that your body is reminded that there is enough food around that it doesn't have to put extra effort into storing it (in the form of body fat). You can do this by making sure that you eat enough food. This is why in the Eat More Diet, I encourage you to eat until you're satisfied. This includes the act of eating. Chewing, tasting, and enjoying your food is also very important. Pay attention to your body. Sense the satisfaction of your hunger. Eat until you're full, but at the same time don't overeat. It's also important to do other things that satisfy your hunger. Chew your food and enjoy the flavor of each mouthful. This will also help to make adaptive thermogenesis work for you and not against you.

2. WHAT YOU EAT: This second way of fueling your Fat Furnace makes use of the "thermic effect of food" which describes the effect of food on metabolic rate. This works thus: Certain foods automatically cause us to burn calories faster or slower, whether or not we're exercising. Step #2 tells you how to use this to help you actually lose weight while you sleep!

STEP #2: USE THE RIGHT FUEL: What we're looking for here is a quick-burning fuel, as opposed to the slow-burning fuels that clog up your machinery and make things run slower. A quick-burning fuel will increase the rate at which your body burns up calories while you're resting. What's the correct fuel to use? There are four different types of fuel from which we derive calories:

I.   Fats, which provide 9 calories per gram.

II.   Carbohydrates, which provide 4 calories per gram. (If carbohydrates are eaten in the form of whole starches such as brown rice, potatoes or whole wheat, the nutrient content is roughly one calorie per gram.)

III. Proteins, which provide 4 calories per gram.

IV.   Alcohol, which provides 7 calories per gram.

In 1982, an experiment was done in Switzerland in which various mixtures of nutrients were used in order to compare the resulting basal metabolic rate, which is the rate at which 'fuel' is burned at rest. (3) Two experimental groups were used. The first group of people were placed on a diet in which the calories were approximately 45 percent carbohydrates, 40 percent fat and 15 percent protein. The second group was placed on a diet in which the calories were approximately 75 percent carbohydrates and 10 percent fats. In this latter study, the protein content was also about 15 percent.

The results were startling! One of their conclusions was that "With the high-carbohydrate low-fat diet, the energy expenditure during sleep was found to be higher than that with the mixed diet." (3) Simply by eating a different mixture of nutrients, the second group showed a remarkable difference in the rate at which calories were burned while they were at rest. The researchers found that those people who were on a high starch diet burned their calories at a significantly higher rate than those who were on the low starch, high fat diet.

This means that the people who were on the high starch diet could lose weight faster or more easily that those on the low starch diet simply because they burned the calories faster! They could either eat the same amount as those on a low starch diet and lose weight faster, or they could eat a little more yet weigh a little less. And they were losing weight while they slept! These were remarkable results!

Following the Eat More Diet shows you how you can make use of the "thermic effect of food" by eating the kinds of foods—high complex carbohydrate foods—to lose weight while you sleep.

3. HOW MUCH YOU PLAY: Playing is the third mechanism to fuel your fat furnace which makes use of the "thermic effect of exercise." Obviously, exercise itself causes us to burn energy. But if you know how to exercise, you can cause your body to increase its metabolic rate even when you are not exercising. (4) Step #3 shows you how.

STEP #3: PLAY, PLAY, PLAY! When, exactly, did exercise become work? Think about it. As a child, you ran and played, and spent all kinds of energy, kept your muscles in tone, kept your cardiovascular system fit, and enjoyed every moment of it! And there's no reason why, now, you can't learn, again, to enjoy exercising. I'll show you how this works in the chapter on that topic. In the meantime, exercise can be play, and you can play off calories as easily as you can work them off. So why not play?

Aerobic exercise is the best kind for dieters. This includes all sorts of fun things, like running, bicycling, skiing, swimming, and a thousand other things you can surely think of. Aerobic exercise allows you to burn calories as well as burn fat! (5) This means exercising at least 30 minutes for a minimum of three to four times per week, and it's even better if you can do it every day. And this kind of exercise does a lot more than burn up calories, though it does that too. But I'm sorry to tell you, the pay-off in calories burnt is rather small. The following list will give you some idea of how inefficient aerobic exercise is with regard to actually getting rid of the calories you so nonchalantly pump into your body:

To Burn:	You Must Run:
One lifesaver	220 yards.
One slice of cheese	1.2 miles.
One apple	1 mile.
A candy bar	2 or more miles.
A hamburger	3 1/2 miles.
A Big burger	6 miles!

**RUNNING ONE MILE BURNS ONLY ABOUT
100 CALORIES!**

It doesn't seem fair, does it?
Why run at all, when the rewards are so small?

The good news is——

Directly burning calories isn't the only benefit. In fact, the
main effect of exercising takes place when we are not exercising at all!

INCREASE YOUR METABOLISM

Let's say that you exercise three to four times per week. This
causes your metabolism to increase at all times. This in turn
means that your basal metabolic rate—the rate at which you
burn calories while you're at rest—increases at all times too, as
a result of the regular exercise. Remarkable, isn't it?

But—sporadic exercise, say once or twice a week, isn't going
to work the miracle. You have to do it regularly, preferably
every day, but at the very least three to four times per week.
This creates what I like to call the "flywheel effect."

HOW MUCH SHOULD I EXERCISE?

FIRST: IF YOU HAVE ANY HEALTH PROBLEMS AT
ALL, SEE YOUR DOCTOR BEFORE DOING ANY
EXERCISES RECOMMENDED IN THIS MANUAL.

One of the best ways to exercise is to choose something that is
fun. Remember, "play your fat away." Personally, I love to
play basketball because it gets me out in the fresh air, I get to
see my friends, and I have a lot of fun. I look forward to it.
It's important to choose something that you like to do because
that's the best way to keep doing it. It could be as simple as
walking around the park with friends or as involved as doing
an Ironman Triathlon. And don't give me age as an excuse
because my radio show co-host, Ruth Heidrich, is 58 years old
and runs the Ironman and 50 other races a year. And her times
are still getting better and better.

One good way to tailor your exercise is to use a simple formula which determines how vigorous your exercise should be to help weight loss. The idea is to get your heart pumping at your "training heart rate" which ensures that your exercise is vigorous enough. *(Again, if you have any health problems or haven't done this in a while, see your doctor before undertaking any exercises in this book.)* Your training heart rate is 60 percent to 80 percent of maximum heart rate. Maximum heart rate is approximately 220 minus your age. Thus the calculation of your training heart rate is as follows.

220 - age = maximum heart rate
maximum heart rate x 60 percent to 80 percent
= training heart rate

Example: for a person age 35 years old,
training heart rate would be 220 - 35 =
185 x .7 = 129
185 x .8 = 148

Thus, optimal exercise occurs when this 35 year-old's heart is beating between 129 beats/minute to 148 beats/minute.

You can check the value of your exercise by counting your pulse against a watch or clock with a second hand.

Then make sure that you exercise at least every other day for at least 30 minutes. A study done at the University of Wisconsin reported in the 1985 issue of the International Journal of Obesity by Dr. D. Lennon and his team of researchers demonstrated that the effect of changing your metabolism *(I call it the "flywheel effect")* takes place if exercise is done on a regular basis at least every other day. (6) Other studies indicate that this is an effective way to help keep your metabolic rate high and the amount of your body fat low. (7,8,9) Remember, what this means is that your metabolic rate gets reset at a higher level and you burn extra calories all the time, even in your sleep!

FINALLY....

Remember that regular physical play or exercise helps you burn calories even when you are not exercising! You're finding your way back to the natural state of human beings, for we all require exercise in order to be healthy, happy—and SLIM!

Besides, we all need a little play now and then.

So why not get started today?

> Play:
> at least 4 times a week
> at least 30 to 40 minutes briskly with
> > a heart rate of at least 60 to 80% of maximum.
> (assuming your doctor says it's OK)

FUELING YOUR FAT FURNACE

Now, if we put these three steps together, we have an excellent formula for beginning success in losing the weight, keeping it off, and enjoying richer vitality and far better health! We have learned to reset our "setpoint" at a higher level, which fires up our "fat furnace," and in this way we are burning calories the easy way, without trying to override our basic biological drives! We are burning calories not only when we are walking, but when we are sitting, working at the desk, reading—and even sleeping! After a while, we're getting rid of fat effortlessly, automatically, without even thinking about it!

And how, again, do you perform this dieting miracle?

Fuel Your Fat Furnace, by:

> I.   Eating enough including chewing and
> savoring your food to satisfaction; no less,
> no more. (Just be sure the foods are high
> EMI foods).

> II.   Eating a high complex carbohydrate diet, and

III.   Playing your fat away with regular physical
        play or exercise 4 times or more per week.

Do these three things and you can begin to "lose weight while
you sleep."

CHAPTER 6

The EMI: A Simple Way to Find Foods That Make You Slim

ACCENTUATE THE POSITIVE

The true treasure to be mined from recent studies on weight loss and dieting is that too much time has been spent emphasizing the negative aspects of weight control. Instead of telling people what they need to do in order to be healthy and slim, most diets concentrate on telling people what not to do. Or, rather, what not to eat. As I've demonstrated with my patients, there is a better way. That's why the Eat More Diet zooms right in on the positive approach, and eliminates the negative. After all, what's the point in knowing what you shouldn't eat, if you don't know what you should eat? Everybody has to eat something!

PRINCIPLES OF THE EAT MORE INDEX

I devised the Eat More Index (EMI) to emphasize the positive and to make it easy for you to find foods that help you be slim. The EMI stands for "Eat More Index". It is actually another name for what I call the "Mass Index" of food because it tells you how much mass or weight a food has for a certain number of calories. It helps you identify the foods you should eat more of to lose weight. The EMI emphasizes what is neglected by most diets by focusing on the mass of food which people eat—and need to eat—rather than just the calorie content of those foods. This helps to identify foods that will fill your stomach and satisfy your hunger while helping you lose weight at the same time.

THE LOGIC OF THE EAT MORE INDEX

An average man or an average active woman requires roughly 2,500 calories per day in order to maintain his or her weight. In order to get 2,500 calories, he or she would have to eat:

30 ears of corn

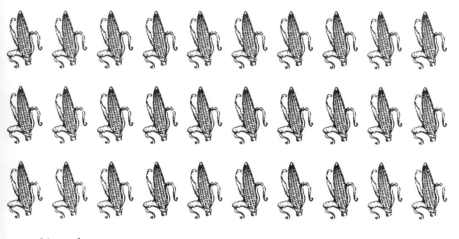

or 31 apples

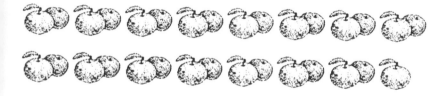

or 24 potatoes

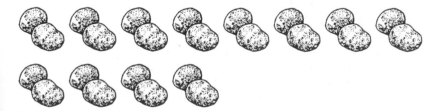

or 17 pounds of broccoli

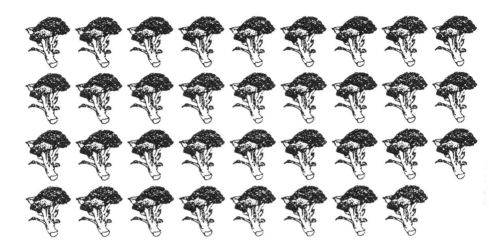

or 2 large burger deluxes with medium fries and a large shake.

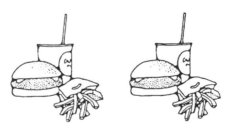

Just about anyone can eat 2 large burgers with fries and a shake in a day with room to spare. This leaves their stomachs partly empty so they want and usually do eat more food, thus exceeding their daily calorie requirement. However, most people can't eat 30 ears of corn, or 31 apples, or 24 potatoes, or 17 pounds of broccoli in a day. Thus, if you eat any of these foods or any combination of these foods until you are satisfied, you will lose weight even though your stomach is full, because it will be less than the amount of food needed to keep your weight. These and many other foods than can help you lose weight can be indentified by the Eat More Index (EMI).

TURNING THE WEIGHT LOSS EQUATION UPSIDE DOWN!

Almost all calorie tables list food as calories per gram or calories per ounce. This means they emphasize calories and tell you to eat less of the high calorie foods. The Eat More Index does just the opposite. IT TURNS THE FOOD-CALORIE EQUATION UPSIDE-DOWN. The Eat More Index (EMI) lists food as grams/calories and then converts it to pounds per 2,500 calories in order to emphasize weight or mass of food, and tells you to EAT MORE of the high EMI foods. The reason it is converted to pounds per 2,500 calories is so that the EMI number represents the number of pounds of a selected food that is required to provide an average day's calories. (An average man or average active woman requires about 2,500 calories per day to maintain his or her weight. Of course individuals vary but 2,500 is used as a simple standard.)

Thus, the Eat More Index number is one that represents generally the number of pounds of a selected food it takes to provide 2500 calories or one day's calorie requirement for an average man or active woman. For example, potatoes have an EMI of 9.4. This means it takes 9.4 pounds of it to make 2500 calories. The black bar graph represents this number. The exception to this rule is in some flour products which do absorb water and provide more satisfaction than is apparent by looking at their dry weight.* This means you can eat these foods and they will help you to lose weight. In fact, any food rated an EMI of 4.1 or more will contribute to weight loss in the average obese individual. A numerical listing of the EMI is also provided if you want to know the actual number of pounds of a selected food required to make 2500 calories.

Along with the EMI value, the EMI chart also indicates the percentage of calories from fat of a selected food. This is represented by the white bar on the EMI chart. This is important because fat is the one category of food you must minimize to lose weight in the long term. It is also important because most

---

* Footnote 1: The one modification I have made in the EMI that does not correspond to the conventional food chart is that I have multiplied certain flour products by a certain factor because they absorb water in the stomach and make the stomach fuller than is apparent by their dry weight. These items are indicated with an asterisk on the EMI charts.

tables only show fat grams. While knowing the amount of fat by grams is important, often the percent fat is disguised in foods that have few calories from protein and carbohydrate. In the EMI chart, the fat percent is clearly designated with the white bar. It is diagrammed with 1 representing 10% and 10 representing 100%. The EMI chart was printed this way to keep the appearance of the chart as simple as possible.

Let's see why high EMI foods make it easier for you to lose weight. Take your average quarter-pound burger with cheese at a fast food restaurant. It would be 630 calories, which is 52% fat and only 261 grams of food. If you eat such oily or fatty foods, you'll fill up about one third of your stomach with those calories of sandwich. If you're dining on two slices of roast beef, you would be getting 594 calories, which is 71% fat and only 170 grams of food. You'll fill your stomach to about one-fourth full with those same 600 calories. But if you eat 600 calories' worth of brown rice—your stomach is completely full!

There's a simple reason it works this way. As it turns out:

- Fats and oils have about 9 calories per gram,
- Protein has about 4 calories per gram,
- Meats have about 5 to 6 calories per gram (because they are a combination of protein and fat),
- Refined carbohydrates have about 4 calories per gram.

On the other hand:

- Whole grains, such as brown rice have less than 1 calorie per gram,
- Broccoli has only 0.3 calories per gram. And so on . . . .

THE SIMPLE MAGIC OF THE EMI: HOW MUCH CAN YOU EAT IN ONE DAY?

Let me illustrate in yet another way why you can eat as much as you want on this diet and still lose weight. Ask yourself:

How much can you eat in one day? Three pounds of food? Four pounds? Five pounds? More?

The studies that we have conducted suggests that in order to stay satisfied, we ordinarily eat somewhere between 3 to 4.1 pounds of solid food per day. (1) An earlier study by another team of researchers suggests that we eat about 2.6 to 4.1 pounds of food to stay satisfied. (2) Of course there is some variation from individual to individual and some variation as a result of differing nutrient content from meal to meal. However, the consistency of these numbers seem to represent a reasonable estimate of what it requires to satisfy the average person.

THE LOGIC OF THE EAT MORE DIET

Now consider that an average man or an average active woman requires about 2,500 calories per day in order to maintain his or her weight according to the RDA estimates. If you were an average man or an average active woman, you would have to eat 9.4 pounds of potatoes every day just to maintain your weight! (Assuming, of course, that potatoes were all you ate.) If you didn't eat that much day after day (and I don't know anyone who can do that), you would lose weight, right? Thus, you can eat as many potatoes as you want and still lose weight.

If you were eating broccoli, you'd have to eat, 17.1 pounds worth (100 cups!) daily. Thus, if you ate potatoes and broccoli as much as you wanted, you would still lose weight. If you were eating just peaches, you'd have to eat 16.5 pounds of them every day to get those 2,500 calories per day just to maintain your present weight. In other words, if you ate all you wanted of potatoes, broccoli, and peaches, it would still be impossible for you to keep from losing weight! And at the same time you'd be eating more food than ever before in your life.

The number to remember is 4.1 for the EMI.

Are you beginning to understand the logic behind the Eat More Diet program? If the maximum amount of food we usually eat per day to satisfy our hunger is about 4.1 pounds, (this varies with your size and your metabolism), then any food that requires more than 4.1 pounds to provide your daily calories will help you lose weight. Potatoes, broccoli, peaches . . . there are hundreds of delicious foods that you can eat all you want of and still lose weight—while getting the proper nutrition! Any combination of these high bulk foods will help you to lose weight, so long as you know which foods they are.

This is where the EMI comes in. With the EMI, you can easily tell which foods are going to contribute to weight loss. It is easy because the EMI is simply the number of pounds* of the selected food it takes to add up to an average day's calorie requirements, about 2,500 calories. In order to lose weight, just keep your food selections to those with an EMI over 4.1. The more you eat of higher EMI foods, the easier it is to lose weight. For example, the broccoli described above has an EMI value of 17.1. In other words, you'd need 17.1 pounds of broccoli to provide 2,500 calories. The EMI of potatoes is 9.4 means you'd need 9.4 pounds of potatoes to get 2,500 calories.

The Eat More Diet emphasizes five aspects of food that will help you lose weight. The EMI chart helps you identify the foods that have these qualities.

1. Maximum Food Mass

Food mass helps you feel full and satisfied. This is why the black bars on the EMI are the most prominent feature of the charts. This black bar represents the satisfaction value of foods by indicating its food mass per calorie—that is how much the food weighs for each calorie. The higher the number, the more you can eat per calorie.

2. Minimum Fat

A major factor in the Eat More Diet is its low fat content. The fat content is indicated by the white bars. Fundamentally, fat is what causes people to be fat and percent fat in the food you eat roughly determines the percent of fat on your body. This

---

* Footnote 1: The one modification I have made in the EMI that does not correspond to the conventional food chart is that I have multiplied certain flour products by a certain factor because they absorb water in the stomach and make the stomach fuller than is apparent by their dry weight. These items are indicated with an asterisk on the EMI charts.

food fat percentage of calories is described by the white bars in the graph. Notice that almost all the food that is high in EMI is very low in fat and vice-versa. While the EMI is a good guideline to low fat foods, it is not foolproof. Some foods that are moderate in EMI are quite high in fat such as avocado and olives. These foods you should not overdo. However, foods that are high in EMI are much better than lower EMI foods with the same fat content because they will satisfy you more.

3.   Maximum Starch

As described in the chapter on how to "Lose weight while you sleep," starch helps you to burn food faster. Foods that are high in starch or complex carbohydrate are generally above 4.1 on the index. The EMI helps you choose these foods. In the next chapter, the inverted pyramid will help you center your diet even more on high complex carbohydrate foods.

4.   Maximum Fiber

Fiber is one of the main substances that makes high EMI foods high in EMI. This is because fiber tends to hold water and does so without calories. In other words, it provides satisfaction without adding weight.

5.   Whole Food

Overall, the EMI encourages you to eat whole food. These are the foods that are naturally high in fiber, low in fat, high in water content, and high in vitamin, mineral, and micronutrient content. For example, you will notice that highly refined foods such as sugar and hard candy are very low on the EMI despite the fact that it has no fat in it. Flour products which are not whole in that they are milled tend to be lower on the EMI than unmilled grain such as brown rice despite the fact that flour products such as breads and noodles are in general quite good because of their low fat high complex carbohydrate qualities. Be careful, however, because flour products such as pastries are laden with fat and sugar and are low on the EMI and will contribute to your weight gain very quickly.

6.   Maximum Micronutrients

Whole foods also contain a wide variety of micronutrients, such as vitamins and minerals. Though we may never completely understand how our bodies utilize all the micronutrients found in whole foods, we do know beyond a doubt that our bodies were designed to use the micronutrients found in natural foods. Recent scientific data increasingly supports the wisdom of eating whole foods because many of the substances found in whole foods may reduce the risk of cancer, heart disease, and help your immune system that is vital to our health. For example, substances such as beta carotene, retinoids, vitamin C, vitamin E and selenium, to name a few, have antioxidant properties that may help prevent cancer. These and so many of the other substances found only in whole foods are essential ingredients in any eating program, if we are ever to function at maximum capacity, ward off disease—and maintain our ideal weight.

The fundamental Eat More Diet principle works for just about anyone. If you eat high EMI foods, primarily whole foods, you'll eat bulkier, more filling foods. You'll feel satisfied, you'll begin to lose weight with no effort other than choosing the right foods, and eventually you'll achieve your ideal weight—without feeling deprived! So the thing to do is focus on changing your foods, rather than driving yourself mad by trying to cut down on the foods you eat. Or, said another way, if you'll just start eating the right foods, you don't have to worry about the amounts you eat. The wizardry of your hunger circuitry will take care of that for you! And that's magic!

CHAPTER 7

Balancing Your Diet With
The Eat More Index (EMI)

More important than the automatic weight loss produced by this diet is the healthfulness of the Eat More Diet. When followed properly, the Eat More Diet is so healthy that not only will it prevent many diseases but it will even reverse many common illnesses. To be sure to reap these benefits, eat a variety of food and follow the Eat More Diet guidelines to food choices. These guidelines help to make your diet similar to that of people who have managed to avoid the high rates of diet-related disease that plagues this nation.

In order to ensure that you are getting the right amount of essential nutrients, it may be useful to look at your food selections from the perspective of a modification of the new food "pyramid" put out by the U.S. Department of Agriculture (USDA). When you're selecting your menus, select items from each of the food groups—as described in the "Modified Pyramid" which I developed for my patients.

THE NEW FOOD GROUPS PYRAMID: A CHANGING CONCEPT

A NEW FOOD GROUPS CHART

In 1992, the Federal Government via the USDA came out with a new food groups chart. It is a new diagram in the shape of a pyramid. I believe that under current circumstances, it is an improvement over the old "four food groups" chart that was recommended in the past. These recommendations are made for the general public and targeted to a large extent at preventing certain deficiency diseases such as iron deficiency and to some extent preventing chronic disease. It is in my opinion and in the opinion of many other scientists still too liberal with dairy and meat groups from the perspective of preventing heart disease and certain cancers.

For those of you who are diligent about your diet, a great deal of medical literature suggests that we can do even better than the food pyramid in terms of maximizing your health with a modified set of recommendations. Note that the recommendations I make here are for motivated individuals such as yourself as opposed to the general public for whom the recommendations in the USDA's pyramid are made. Thus, in the Eat More Diet, I like to use a modified "inverted pyramid" which I believe will provide better protection against the diseases that are the leading causes of death of Americans than the existing pyramid.

UNDERSTAND THE FOOD PYRAMID

The food guide pyramid is a diagram which provides a way to help you ensure that the nutrients you obtain from food is adequate. Basically, the USDA pyramid (1) tells us to eat on a daily basis the following:

Grains:	6-11 Servings
Vegetables:	3-5 Servings
Fruit:	2-4 Servings
Dairy:	2-3 Servings
Meat/Beans:	2-3 Servings
Fats/Oils/Sweets:	Sparingly

WHAT IS A "SERVING"?

A "serving" is what an average person might serve of a selected food at a single sitting. This is actually somewhat arbitrary because how much a person may serve of certain foods varies a great deal. Nonetheless, it provides a starting point. Here are examples of "servings".

Food Guide Pyramid
A Guide to Daily Food Choices

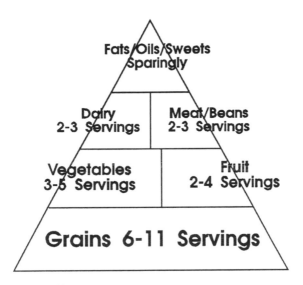

USDA 1992

The USDA's Food Guide Pyramid is an improvement over the old "four food groups" concept as a recommendation for the general public. However, for optimal health for most motivated adults, the "Inverted Pyramid" (to follow) is even better.

Cereal grains group:
   1/2 C cooked cereal, pasta, or brown rice,
   1 slice of bread, or 1 oz ready-to-eat cereal

Vegetables group:
   1 C raw leafy greens, 1/2 C cooked,
   chopped, raw or other vegetables.

Fruit group:
   1 medium fruit, 1/2 C chopped,
   cooked or canned fruit

Dairy group:
   1 C milk, yogurt or ice cream, 1-1/2 oz cheese,
   or 2 oz processed cheese

Beans, fish, poultry, meat group:
   1/2 C cooked beans, 2-3 oz cooked fish,
   chicken, or meat, 1 egg.

The modified "Inverted Food Pyramid" that I designed is slightly different. I recommend the following for daily use:

Whole Grains:	8-13 Servings
Vegetables:	3-5 Servings
Fruit:	2-4 Servings
Non-Dairy Calcium Foods:	2-3 Servings
Non-Cholesterol Protein/Iron Foods:	2-3 Servings

And for optional or special occasion use:

Dairy (which is an extension of the calcium group)
Fish/Poultry/Meat
Fats/Oils/Sugar

Notice the changes in the pyramid. I have made the fats/oils/sugar section smaller and minimized the dairy and meat foods and moved them downward into the bottom of the Inverted Food Pyramid as optional/occasional foods. In place of the dairy group, I have created a non-dairy calcium group and in place of the meat group I have created a non-cholesterol protein/iron group. Notice also, that the Inverted Food

Dr. Shintani's Inverted Food Pyramid

A Guide to Daily Food Choices

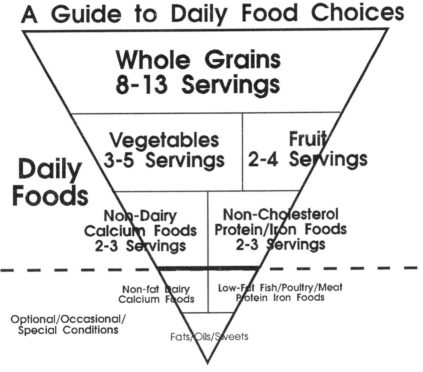

**Whole Grains
8-13 Servings**

Daily Foods

**Vegetables
3-5 Servings**

**Fruit
2-4 Servings**

**Non-Dairy
Calcium Foods
2-3 Servings**

**Non-Cholesterol
Protein/Iron Foods
2-3 Servings**

Non-fat Dairy
Calcium Foods

Low-Fat Fish/Poultry/Meat
Protein Iron Foods

Optional/Occasional/
Special Conditions

Fats/Oils/Sweets

(c) Shintani 1992

Pyramid is separated by a dotted line at the apex. These foods are optional and for special occasions or certain health conditions only. This reflects the fact that these foods were not eaten on a daily basis in populations such as Mediterranean and Asian populations that rarely suffer from the diseases that plague us today such as heart disease. It also reflects modern literature that indicates that a vegetarian diet can be as healthy or healthier than a diet with daily animal product consumption. (2)

THE WHOLE GRAIN GROUP (STARCHES)

We should get used to the idea of whole grain as our main dish. Most of the world and humanity throughout history did. This is why I inverted the pyramid and placed this most important group at the top. In fact, for most people, at least 50 percent of your meal should come from this group of foods. This reflects the fact that whole grains were the center of the diet of populations throughout history and around the world before modernization of their diets and before they were dying of the diseases that kill us today. For example, the staple food of most of the world is rice when you consider that this is the chief food of China, India, Japan, and Southeast Asia. The staple of the Americas was corn, and the staple of Europe was wheat and rye. In Polynesia, the main food was taro, a starchy potato-like root.

If you look at the EMI, you will notice that whole grains and starchy foods are medium on the EMI. Remember that the EMI number represents the number of pounds of a selected food it takes to provide an 2,500 calories, roughly an average day's calories for an average active woman or an average sedentary man.

For example:

Food	EMI	Pounds to make 2500 calories
Brown rice	4.59	4.59
Corn	6.50	6.50
Pasta	4.14	4.14
Potatoes	9.58	9.58

As I discussed above, this is ideal because eating mainly high EMI foods would cause you to not get enough calories and eating mainly low EMI foods would cause you to get too much *(the way we are in America now)*. While many of the familiar foods from the cereal group are refined products, such as breads and pastas, you will notice that these refined complex carbohydrates are lower on the EMI and thus not as good for weight loss.

In this group, whole grains tend to be higher in EMI and thus better for weight loss. Thus, the type of cereal grain you should eat in order to maximize the Eat More Diet principles are unprocessed whole grains, such as brown rice, corn, oatmeal, barley, and other unrefined grains. The next best would be flour products made from whole grains such as whole wheat bread, whole grain noodles, and whole wheat tortillas. The least desirable would be flour products made from refined grains such as white bread and white noodles. In any case, remember to use the cereal grain group as the basis for your diet, then round out your menu with foods from the other groups.

THE VEGETABLE AND FRUIT GROUPS

After you've selected your main dish, your whole starch, you should fill up on the vegetable and fruit group. This group has the foods that are highest on the EMI. Approximately 25 to 30 percent of your calories should come from a variety of vegetables and fruit. The USDA recommends 3-5 servings of vegetables and 2-4 servings of fruit. I recommend a similar amount. You must EAT MORE of this group than you are accustomed to obtain an adequate amount. Eating high EMI vegetables help contribute to your health, weight loss and food satisfaction. At the same time you will be getting a nice selection of vitamins, minerals and micronutrients at the cost of very few calories.

Examples of vegetables:

Food	EMI	Pounds to make 2500 calories
Kale	10.3	10.3
Bean Sprouts	11.9	11.9
Carrots	13.0	13.0
Onions	14.8	14.8
Pumpkin	16.6	16.6
Broccoli	17.1	17.1
Cabbage	22.8	22.8
Zucchini	32.1	32.1

Examples of fruit:

Food	EMI	Pounds to make 2500 calories
Banana	6.43	6.43
Apples	9.42	9.42
Oranges	15.60	15.60
Watermelon	21.00	21.00
Grapefruit	27.30	27.30

One word of caution. Do not go overboard on eating fruit, especially dried fruit. For most individuals, an excess of fruit sugar—which is plentiful in most fruit—makes it difficult to lose weight. In many individuals, it can cause a rise in triglycerides, a co-risk-factor for heart disease (along with cholesterol).

THE NON-DAIRY CALCIUM GROUP
(Instead of the Dairy Group)

Why The Calcium Group?

Why have I changed this group in the Inverted Pyramid from the "dairy group" to the "calcium group"? I call this the non-dairy calcium group rather than the dairy group because it focuses attention on the real health issue behind this food group, calcium. Because most dairy foods are high in fat and have low EMI values, I have moved the dairy group in with the optional/occasional food category in the pyramid.

Why does this group focus on calcium? Ever see a person in their later years hunched over as if they couldn't stand straight? It happens more in women than in men. This condition is known as osteoporosis which is the result of the thinning of bones due to the gradual loss of calcium. This is why the calcium group is important. Eating foods that contain enough calcium helps to prevent osteoporosis. But it is becoming apparent that there are many factors besides calcium that help cause and prevent osteoporosis. (4) Some of these factors that promote osteoporosis includes the following:

- Excessive Protein Intake
- Lack of Exercise
- Smoking
- Estrogen Imbalance
- Lack of Vitamin D
- Excessive Intake of Phosphorus
- Caffeine
- Sodium

While it makes some sense to eat more calcium to avoid osteoporosis, it is time we considered all factors, not just one. Perhaps one of the most important things to consider is the impact of excessive intake of foods that might be recommended in order to provide calcium. Dairy food, especially, has been propagandized into the American diet, as "man's perfect food." Actually it is baby cow's "perfect food" and not "man's." Most dairy foods are so high in fat and cholesterol that most well-informed nutritionists now recommend that we substantially reduce our intake of whole dairy food, and if it is eaten at all, to use the very low fat or no-fat variety such as skim-milk. This is because fat and cholesterol are related to heart disease and cancer.

And frankly, there are far less hazardous sources of calcium. We do not have to ingest the cholesterol and high fat in order to get our daily allowances of calcium. Greens are a great source of calcium. Kale, collard greens, and broccoli are excellent sources of calcium, and none of them contain the fats and cholesterol that contribute to heart disease, cancer and other illnesses. *(Spinach does have a lot of oxalate that makes much of the calcium hard to absorb.)* Calcium is the primary nutrient in dairy foods that has long been the justification for keeping the "dairy" food group as one of the essentials in the old four food groups and now in the USDA "Food Guide Pyramid". Therefore, why not call this food group the `calcium group' so that these other safer sources of calcium are not overlooked?

Calcium Density in Selected Food
For weight control,
dairy is not the best source of calcium

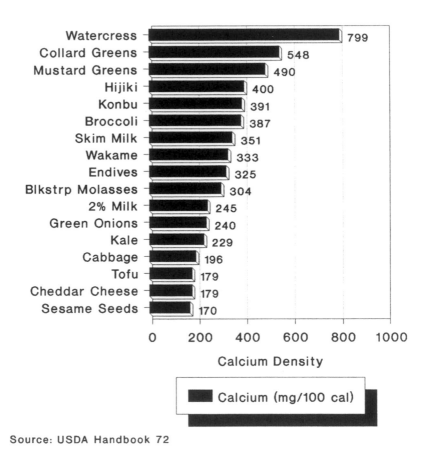

Source: USDA Handbook 72

For example:

1 Cup of whole milk (244 g)	= 288 mg calcium	150 cal
1 Ounce Cheddar cheese (28.4 Gm)	= 204 mg calcium	114 cal
1 Spear of broccoli (190 g)	= 205 mg calcium	50 cal
1 Cup of collards (190 g)	= 148 mg calcium	25 cal
1 Cup of kelp seaweed (konbu) (185 g)	= 317 mg calcium	60 cal
1 Cup of turnip greens (144 g)	= 197 mg calcium	30 cal

Then, look at the EMI value of these foods and see which ones calorie for calorie satisfy you the most.

Food	EMI	Pounds to make 2500 cal
Cheddar cheese	1.37	1.37
Broccoli	17.1	17.1
Collard greens	12.1	12.1
Kelp (Konbu)	12.7	12.7
Turnip greens	27.3	27.3

(Note that the EMI chart does not work with beverages [e.g. milk] because the fluid in beverages overstates the EMI value. In addition, on the Eat More Diet, I don't recommend the use of any calorie-containing beverages because they may provide a great deal of calories and have poor satisfaction value as compared to whole food.)

You can see that from the perspective of weight loss, the cheese which seems like a good source of calcium is actually not as good as high calcium greens and seaweeds. Another way to look at calcium in order to determine the best source from the perspective of weight loss is calcium density. This gives you the amount of calcium per calorie of food. Once again, you can see from the following chart that dairy is not the best source of calcium.

If you want to look at calcium while you are trying to lose weight, you might even look at it in terms of mg per CALORIE instead of mg per cup. In other words, how much calcium you get for each calorie of food you take in. This way, you get the

CHOLESTEROL
What is one simple rule you can use to find cholesterol in your food?

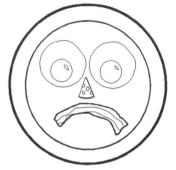

Anything that has a face on it has cholesterol in it.

This includes foods such as beef, pork, chicken, fish, shrimp, and foods that come from things with faces such as eggs and cheese. There is no cholesterol in plant-based foods such as grains, beans, vegetables, and fruit.

CHOLESTEROL IN FOODS
Why do they recommend chicken and fish?
Cholesterol content in 3-1/2 oz of food

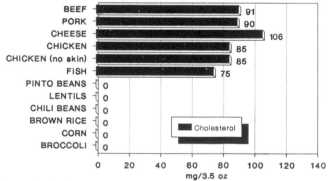

The reason is that fat content is lower in chicken and fish. However, cholesterol content is high in these foods even if you remove the skin.

most calcium for the least number of calories. You'll find an interesting change in what are the best sources of calcium if you look at it in this way. You'll find that greens and sea vegetables turn out to be the best.

From the perspective of the EMI, you will see that dairy foods are low on the EMI and considered fat foods—in that they contain fat, but also in that they help make you and keep you fat. There are many other foods, on the other hand, that contain all and more of the essential nutrients that dairy contains, yet are high on the index—therefore, they help you lose weight and maintain that weight loss. These high-calcium foods are mostly greens, the same foods from which the cows get their calcium to begin with! So why not get the calcium straight from the source.

As for dairy foods I have placed them in the "optional/occasional" group as a smaller part of the diet to be consistent with the idea that this is NOT a required food and certainly not the optimal daily food for most adults. I have placed it in a position adjacent to the non-dairy calcium group to show that it is a source of calcium.

THE PROTEIN/IRON GROUP (Instead of the meat group)

The "meat group" is also misunderstood. As I described above, advertising would have you believe that this is solely a "meat" group. But contrary to this highly promoted notion, most dietitians know that legumes or beans are intended to be included in this group. If you look at the EMI of meat, fish, poultry and beans, the items that are highest on the index are the beans and legumes. Thus, the best sources of protein from the perspective of weight loss are beans, and not meats.

In fact, even from the perspective of good health, beans are better than any animal food because of the absence of cholesterol in beans, and anything that comes from something with a face on it has cholesterol in it. Nothing of plant origin does. This means that in order to protect yourself from heart disease, it is better to eat beans than beef. This is why meats, poultry, and fish have been placed in the optional/occasional category of the Modified Pyramid. In addition, if you look at the fat

PROTEIN AND AMINO ACID TABLE

Essential Amino Acids (in Mg) Available in 2,200 Cal of Food (RDA for adult female)

Food	PROTEIN	TRYPTO	THREO	ISOLEU	LEUCINE	LYSINE	METHIO	PHENYL	VALINE
RDA Female	50	250	450	650	950	800	425	475	650
Rice, Brown	51	714	2130	2465	4815	2222	1308	3009	3414
Corn	73	542	3072	3072	8312	3283	1596	3584	4427
Potato	46	776	1810	2047	2995	3017	776	2279	2801
Turnip	86	982	2768	4018	3661	3929	1250	1964	3214
Kale	110	1829	6768	9023	10548	9023	1402	7682	8231
Broccoli	220	2608	8151	9782	11738	12716	3043	7608	11520
Beans, Kidney	129	1467	6846	8976	13583	11736	1576	8726	9584
Beef	132	1994	7798	8016	14098	14838	4568	6965	8673
Cheese, Cheddar	179	1993	5497	9593	14805	12878	4052	8147	10316
Rice, White	47	590	1809	2173	4170	1821	1181	1688	3077

content, it is clear that the fat content of beans are the lowest of the protein sources though the amount of protein is very similar.

For example:

3 oz of lean hamburger	= 21 g protein
3 oz lean and fat pot roast	= 17 g protein
3 oz broiled steak	= 20 g protein
3 oz chicken	= 20 g protein
1 pork chop	= 16 g protein

And:

1 Cup lima beans	= 16 g protein
1 Cup split peas, cooked	= 16 g protein
1 Cup garbanzo beans, cooked	= 15 g protein

Not much difference in the protein content, but a world of difference in its health and weight loss value! Just look at the EMI for protein-containing foods. You will see that beans and legumes are best for weight loss because they fill you up more per calorie.

Food	EMI	Pounds of food to make 2500 cal
Hamburger	1.88	1.88
Roast beef	1.16	1.16
Pork chop	2.09	2.09
Lima beans	4.92	4.92
Split peas	6.5	6.5
Garbanzo beans	5.58	5.58

THE PROTEIN MYTH

Furthermore, the emphasis on protein is actually unnecessary for most of us as we in America generally eat too much protein. The only people who get inadequate protein are those who can't get enough food, and those who eat too many "empty calories" such as in the form of alcohol, fat, and sugar. In fact, excessive protein can be harmful, not only from the perspective of osteoporosis as discussed above, (3) but also from the perspective of kidney disease. The problem is even worse if the

Iron Density in Selected Foods
For weight control,
beef is not the best source of iron

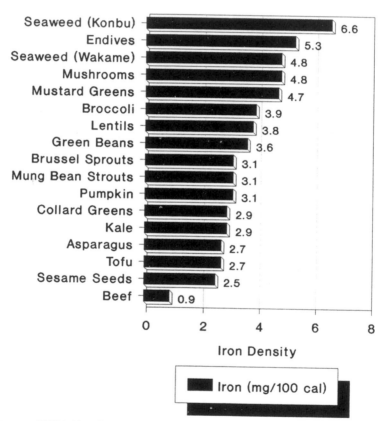

Food	Iron Density
Seaweed (Konbu)	6.6
Endives	5.3
Seaweed (Wakame)	4.8
Mushrooms	4.8
Mustard Greens	4.7
Broccoli	3.9
Lentils	3.8
Green Beans	3.6
Brussel Sprouts	3.1
Mung Bean Strouts	3.1
Pumpkin	3.1
Collard Greens	2.9
Kale	2.9
Asparagus	2.7
Tofu	2.7
Sesame Seeds	2.5
Beef	0.9

Iron Density

Iron (mg/100 cal)

Source: USDA Handbook 72

protein source is from animal proteins which have been associated with certain kinds of cancer.

One of the myths about protein is that grains, beans and vegetables are somehow inadequate sources of protein and that there must be careful combining. If you look at the chart below, you will see that even if you took a single so-called "incomplete protein" food and ate a whole day's worth of calories (in this example 2200 calories which is the RDA for a 25 to 50 year-old woman), of this food without combining it with any other, none of the examples demonstrate any deficiency of any essential amino acid! In fact, most of the amino acids are present in great excess. And in the case of beef and cheese, these foods contain more than 1000% the RDA of methionine, the sulfur-containing amino acid. Sulfur-containing amino-acids are the ones implicated in causing a loss of calcium in the urine which could promote osteoporosis.

As for total protein, just about all the grains and vegetables exceed the RDA total protein content, and they all have more than 75% the RDA which is recognized as safe provided the amino acid mix is adequate. Even white rice has nearly the RDA for protein, and meets the RDA for all essential amino acids.

WHAT ABOUT IRON?

Iron, of course, is important in the making of red blood cells. Red blood cells are necessary to carry oxygen to all parts of our bodies. If we don't have enough iron, not enough blood cells are made and we wind up with a condition known as "iron deficiency anemia." The "meat" group has been considered to be important in that this group of foods is supposed to provide a good supply of this nutrient. However, once again, if we're trying to lose weight, let's look at iron sources from the perspective of how much iron there is per calorie. As in calcium, we want to get as much iron as we can per calorie so that we don't gain weight trying to get enough iron.

As for animal food I have placed it in the "optional/occasional" group as a smaller part of the diet to be consistent with the idea that this is NOT a required food and certainly not the optimal daily food for most adults. I have placed it in a position adjacent to the non-cholesterol protein-iron group to show that it is a source of protein and iron.

OPTIONAL FOODS

The final piece of the pyramid is the optional foods group. I have placed the dairy foods and meat/poultry/fish foods in this category along with the fats, oils and sweets. Notice that I have placed this at the bottom of the Inverted Pyramid and separated it from the rest of the food groups. Nearly all of us can get along fine without these foods and be all the healthier for it. We certainly do not need them on a daily basis. This is why I have classified these foods as "optional, special occasion, and special condition" foods. In addition, these foods you will see all have a very low EMI value and will easily begin to scuttle any diet. The foods are low in bulk value and will not provide the satisfaction value of a high EMI food and will induce the consumption of more calories. Moreover, they are for the most part high in fat which will help you gain weight in your sleep and promote the production of more body fat.

For those who are not on an ideal diet, or who have some health conditions that affect their digestion, absorption, metabolism or otherwise affect their nutrition, these foods may be appropriate.

ABOUT ANIMAL FOOD (Meat/Poultry/Fish)

You may notice that there are no foods of animal origin in the recipes in this book. Frankly, one of the reasons for this is that I don't know how to cook using such foods (and I don't intend to learn how). This is a personal choice and I don't believe in imposing my personal choice on others. However, I believe that there is so much pressure on people to eat foods of flesh origin (how many fast food commercials have you seen lately?) that we don't need to learn more ways to do this anyway.

As for weight loss and the EAT MORE DIET approach, it can be done with or without flesh foods. Whatever your choice may be, however, remember that almost all animal foods are low EMI foods and tend to make you fat. Almost all high EMI foods and almost all moderate EMI foods are of vegetable origin. Thus, learning to use and enjoy these vegetable, grain, and fruit foods are indispensable to losing weight in the long run. I can recall Dr. William Castelli, director of the most famous heart study in the world, the Framingham Heart Study saying that "the best way to avoid heart disease is to learn 10 good recipes and use them all the time." I hope that you can consider this suggestion and replace most if not all of your recipes with the high EMI meals found in this book.

If you use animal type foods, notice that they are low on the EMI and must be limited to small amounts and only on occasion. Use the EMI and make your choices with this in mind. The only foods from this group that are reasonable are foods for the Eat More Diet are foods such as low fat fish, shrimp, lobster, and crab, and some cuts of skinless poultry. Remember that these foods are high in cholesterol and can contribute to heart disease.

Remember that our ancestors didn't eat flesh most of the time. The reason we know this is that there were no refrigerators a century ago and during the entire prior existence of humanity. This means that meat, fish, chicken, and dairy food would have spoiled in a short while and could not be eaten daily. This is one of the reasons there was little obesity and heart disease back then.

Remember that if you eat a great deal of protein, especially animal protein, you may need additional calcium to counteract the calcium-wasting effect of the high protein content of your meat, fish, or chicken meal. There are many supplements that will do fine and if you use dairy foods, use only skim milk and skim milk products.

ABOUT DAIRY FOODS

The Eat More Diet places dairy foods in the optional/occasional category because in general, most dairy foods are high in EMI and contribute to weight gain, and contain too much cholesterol and fat. Those that are low in fat such as skim milk are considered calorie-containing beverages which may not support weight loss as I describe at the end of this chapter.

In addition to the problem of diseases caused by too much cholesterol and fat with which dairy food may be linked, milk protein allergy is one of the most common food allergies known in the United States. And when we look at diet from a global perspective, dairy as an essential food makes no sense. It couldn't possibly be "man's perfect food." I say this because roughly 70 percent of the world's people are lactose intolerant as adults. *(Lactose is a form of milk sugar.)* They feel gassy, bloated and even have diarrhea when milk is ingested. This is because most people in the world do not have enough of an enzyme known as lactase to break down the lactose in their stomachs. The only living things that cow's milk is the perfect for is baby cows!

More recently a study from Norway indicated that dairy food consumption is correlated with the incidence of juvenile onset diabetes, (5) and the American Pediatrics Association no longer recommends whole cow's milk for infants under 9 months because it can cause anemia. (6)

In fact, it is rapidly becoming evident that one of the only redeeming qualities of dairy food in a well nourished society is its calcium content. Even this concept of using milk as a source of calcium is being questioned by some scientists. Consider, for a moment, that billions of people never take any dairy food as adults and yet live healthy, osteoporosis-free lives. A good example of this is found in the now famous "China diet" study wherein Chinese populations were studied and the researchers found almost no osteoporosis — despite the complete absence of dairy food in the diets of the adults. (7)

The question about the value of dairy food in preventing osteoporosis particularly because of its high protein content led one researcher to state that:

"Over the years, doubts have arisen concerning the use of milk as a calcium source in the prevention of osteoporosis, particularly because of potential offsetting effects of protein and phosphorus." (8)

Another distinguished researcher in his summary of a 1988 international congress meeting on nutrition and vegetarian diets stated:

> "Given that a majority of Americans (including vegetarians) consume excessive amounts of protein, a reduction to a lower level might be an important consideration in the prevention of calcium loss . . ." (9)

If you choose to use dairy, remember to use it like a supplement, and not a daily food. Use it if you are not getting adequate calcium from greens or are eating too much protein. And if you do use dairy food, use skim milk products to minimize the effect on weight retention and health.

ABOUT FATS/OILS/SUGARS.

Fats/Oils/Sugars are the category of food in the apex of the USDA pyramid as well as the modified pyramid. The USDA recommendations for the general public is to use these foods sparingly. In the modified pyramid, my recommendations for healthy adult individuals wanting to lose weight is to use these foods "optionally or occasionally". The reason for this is that these are the foods that are lowest on the EMI and can easily turn a weight-loss food into a weight-gain food.

Oils

Included in the fats and oils category are foods such as:
        Lard
        Vegetable oil
        Shortening
        Butter
        Margarine
        Mayonnaise
        Salad Dressing (except no-oil dressings)

It doesn't matter whether the food item is from plant or animal sources in terms of its effect on weight. Both plant and animal fats are 9 calories per gram and both will make you fat. Neither does it matter whether it says "no-cholesterol" or "cholesterol free" because cholesterol has no calories and thus has no effect on weight gain or loss. (It will increase the risk of heart disease, however).

SLIM PIE
Food Choices in Approximate Proportions
Based on the Inverted Pyramid

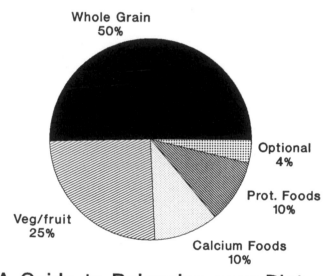

Whole Grain
50%

Optional
4%

Prot. Foods
10%

Veg/fruit
25%

Calcium Foods
10%

A Guide to Balancing your Diet
(Preferrably Whole, Fresh Foods)

Individual needs may vary
(c) Shintani 1992

Sugars

Included in the sugars category are foods such as:
> White sugar
> Brown sugar
> Honey
> Molasses
> Maple Syrup
> Rice Syrup
> Candy

These foods are not as bad as the fats and oil in terms of weight loss because they contain little or no fat. However, their EMI value is low (around 1.4) and despite being low in fat can still make you fat. This is a pitfall of diets that only consider fat grams and ignore the bulk value of foods. For example, I have seen patients eating a lot of jelly beans on a simple fat gram diet because such a diet allows unlimited amounts of non-fat foods. Unfortunately, these individuals lost no weight because it was easy to get a lot of calories and sabotage their diet with foods such as jelly beans which are low EMI foods. An additional problem with sugars is that they are empty calories and may cause a deprivation of vitamins and minerals.

In using sugars, I prefer to use items such as blackstrap molasses which is high in calcium or syrups such as maple or rice syrup which have some starch in them.

SLIM PIE

For those of you who like pie charts, consider this chart which I call "slim pie." It is roughly a representation of the recommendations which I make in the inverted pyramid. I present it in this form because for some people it is easier to look at their meals in terms of percentage than in terms of servings.

FOR VEGETARIANS

If you choose to eliminate the optional part of the pyramid, you will have a vegetarian diet. This is in some ways an ideal diet if done carefully. Indeed the original diet of humanity according to the Bible in the book of Genesis was vegetarian. Such diets have been followed with great success by many people in this country and many other countries. The Seventh Day Adventists are a group who have practiced vegetarianism for many years and have demonstrated superior health to that of the general population. (2) Saints and holy people around the world throughout history have also done well with a vegetarian diet. Monks in China and Japan have used a vegetarian approach to healing the illnesses of many people. There are great moral, spiritual, and even environmental reasons to do so. I hope that everyone will educate themselves about these reasons and make choices about their diet based on this knowledge. These reasons aside, however, I hope you will realize that more and more scientists are recognizing the value of a vegetarian diet or a near-vegetarian diet in the maintenance of good health.

A well respected nutrition researcher, pointed out that:

> "Regardless of whether people choose vegetarian or non-vegetarian patterns with sound nutritional planning, they can reap health benefits."
> (11)

EXAMPLES OF FOODS FROM THE INVERTED PYRAMID

The following foods are intended as examples and not as a complete list of foods. There are literally thousands of other foods to choose from.

GRAINS

Unlimited use	Moderate use	Rare use
Brown Rice	Whole Wheat Bread	White Bread
Corn	Whole Wheat Pasta	White Flour Pasta
Barley	Whole Wheat Pita Bread	White Flour Tortillas
Millet	Whole Wheat Chapati	White Flour Bagels
Whole Oats	Whole Wheat Bagels	While Flour Muffins
Buckwheat	Whole Wheat Muffins	While Flour Noodles
Wheat Berries	Buckwheat Noodles	
Potatoes	Instant Oatmeal	
Taro	White Rice	
Poi	Corn Tortillas	

VEGETABLE GROUP

Unlimited use	**Rare Use**
Kale	Avocado
Collard Greens	Olives
Broccoli	
Turnips	
Chinese Cabbage	
Cabbage	
Carrots	
Onions	
Pumpkin	
Squash	
Radish	
Cucumber	
Celery	
Swiss Chard	
Cauliflower	
Artichokes	
Asparagus	
Zucchini	
Tomatoes	
Watercress	
Brussels Sprouts	
Burdock root	
Lotus Root	
Spinach	
Green Onion	

FRUIT GROUP

Moderate Use

Apples	Grapefruits
Apricot	Cherries
Banana	Raspberries
Plums	Blueberries
Pears	Melons
Nectarines	Cantaloupes
Grapes Oranges	Tangerines
Peaches	Lemons
Strawberries	

NON-DAIRY CALCIUM GROUP

Unlimited use	Occasional Use
Kale	Tofu
Collard Greens	Tofu products
Konbu (seaweed)	Blackstrap molasses
Hijiki (seaweed)	Sesame seeds
Wakame (seaweed)	
Broccoli	
Mustard Greens	
Endives	
Chinese Cabbage	
Watercress	
Spinach	
Green Onion	
Brussels Sprouts	
Amaranth	

NON-ANIMAL PROTEIN/IRON GROUP

Unlimited use		Moderate Use
Kale	Green Beans	Peanuts
Konbu	Endives	Cashews
Hijiki	Lima Beans	Sunflower seeds
Wakame	Lentils	Sesame seeds
Broccoli	Garbanzo Beans	Soy Beans
Brussels Sprouts	Green Beans	
Mustard Greens		

OPTIONAL/OCCASIONAL FOODS

Remember that almost all the foods in these categories are low on the EMI and will likely contribute to weight gain. If you use them, use the lowest fat or no fat varieties.

MEAT	DAIRY
Beef	Cheese
Pork	Milk
Chicken	Yogurt
Fish	Cottage Cheese
Turkey	Cream Cheese
Hamburger	Cream
(and all other flesh	Eggs
containing products)	

FATS/OILS/SUGAR

Fats & Oils	Sugars
Lard	White sugar
Vegetable oil	Brown sugar
Shortening	Honey
Butter	Molasses
Margarine	Maple Syrup
Mayonnaise	Rice Syrup
Salad Dressing (except no-oil dressings)	Candy
Pastries	

ABOUT BEVERAGES

The best beverage for all of us is pure water. I can't emphasize that enough. Drinking water or other non-caloric beverages with such as herb teas and sparkling water will actually help you in your effort to lose excess fat. I also prefer the beverages to have no caffeine or artificial sweeteners in them.

You will notice that beverages are not on the EMI. There are two reasons for this. First, I don't recommend the use of beverages that contain calories such as liquors, soft drinks, milk, milk shakes, even juices. Part of the reasoning for this is that in many populations that remained slim all their lives, beverages containing calories were not used very often. They used water or herb teas instead.

The second reason is that not much is known about the impact of calorie-containing beverages on weight gain or loss. We do know that drinking beverages that contain calories means very little if any fiber content and requires no chewing so that the satisfaction level is less that by eating a whole food. It is easy to drink the calories of an orange in the form of orange juice in a matter of seconds where it would take a lot more time, chewing and swallowing to eat a whole orange. The act of eating, chewing and swallowing are important in the satisfaction of hunger. In addition, studies comparing the consumption of apple juice to apple sauce to whole apples, indicate that the blood sugar response is most extreme in apple juice. Because blood sugar levels have some impact on hunger and satiety, we may conclude that the apple is better than the juice in terms of inducing satisfaction and long term weight loss.

If you choose to drink beverages with calories in them, choose fruit juices with no added sugar. If you choose dairy, select only skim milk. But always remember that the best beverage is pure water.

USING THE EMI TO UNLOCK THE SECRET TO DIETING

Let's now look at how the principles of the Eat More Diet help you to understand how some other diets work and how you can design a balanced weight loss diet of your own. The Eat More Index provides the key that unlocks the secret to many diets that have been successful in causing weight loss. Many of these diets have been focused on a single food or a small number of foods and boasted that no calorie restriction was required. For example, the "grapefruit diet" that was popular many years ago basically told you to eat only grapefruits in the initial stages of the diet.

The following are some examples of weight loss diets that have used this limited food choice approach. I am using these as examples so that you understand how to use the EMI.

Grapefruit Diet

A good example of a single-food diet is a diet based on grapefruit. I don't recommend such a diet because obviously it is not balanced, but some people use "fruit only" days to help with weight loss. This type of diet was popular many years ago and was based on the simple rule of eating nothing but grapefruit for a period of time. Some proponents suggested that weight loss was due to "enzymes" in grapefruit that "melted" your fat. The truth of the matter is that enzymes in food don't get absorbed as enzymes (they are broken down in the intestines and absorbed as amino acids and peptides) and never have an opportunity to work on your body fat.

The real reason this diet works can be found through the use of the Eat More Index (EMI). Look at the Index and you will see that the EMI of grapefruit is 27.4 which means that it takes 27.4 pounds of grapefruit to make 2500 calories. There is no way that anyone is going to eat 27.4 pounds of grapefruit in a day. Thus, no matter if calories were never counted or that the enzymes don't work the way they purportedly work, this would cause automatic weight loss. I don't recommend this approach because of its lack of variety and balance but it does work and it illustrates the principle behind the Eat More Diet and the EMI.

Rice Diet

One of the best scientifically documented diet is one based on rice. (12) First tested in 1939, rice was effectively used as the initial phase of a diet to lower blood pressure. In this phase, white rice and fruit are used as the exclusive food in the diet, and no salt was permitted. For example, such a diet would include:

Breakfast	Lunch	Dinner
1 multi-vitamin		
1 Fruit	2 Fruit	2 Fruit
1/2 C rice	1 C rice	2 C rice

If you look at the EMI number of these foods, you would find that white rice has an EMI of 5.01. In other words it requires 5.01 pounds in order to make 2500 calories. Now, you know that people just won't eat that much rice in a day. As for the fruit, if you eat apples, the EMI number is 9.42 and thus, it would take 9.42 pounds of apples (31 of them) to make your day's 2500 calories. Obviously, no matter how much you ate, you would be full far before you reached the amount of calories you needed to keep your weight on. Thus, this type of diet caused weight loss because of the high EMI values of the foods used. However, it is not practical to stay on such a diet for a long period of time because it will not provide you with a good balance of nutrients. In fact the proponents of this diet recognize this and thus recommend a multi-vitamin be taken daily to make up for the deficiencies of such a diet.

Your Designer Diet: Using the EMI to Custom-Design your Diet

With the EMI, you can create your own "Designer diet" if you wish, and you can make it one that you can stay on safely for good. Just remember that in using the EMI, the important number to remember is 4.1. That is, you should eat only foods that are higher than 4.1 on the EMI. The reason I use this number as a guideline is that satiety studies have shown that this is around the upper limit of the number of pounds of food an average person eats in a day to be satisfied. All you have to do is pick a combination of high EMI foods that are higher than 4.1, and eat as much of these foods as you want in order to satisfy your hunger. Balance your diet with the "Inverted Pyramid" by picking foods that fit the pyramid. If you want to keep it really simple, just pick a few foods that fit the categories and repeat these foods for a short period of time. For best initial results, do not use any foods in the optional bottom part of the pyramid.

Here is an example of a simple diet similar to the above diets but based on the EMI. Choose brown rice to serve as your whole grain, broccoli can serve as your vegetable, high iron food, and high calcium food, and apples can serve as your fruit.

For your whole grain choose oatmeal, brown rice and baked potato. For your vegetable, choose carrots and zucchini. For your fruit, choose grapefruit and apple, for your high calcium food choose broccoli and kale, and for your high protein food, the savory beans suffice.

BREAKFAST

1 C Oatmeal	EMI = 9.9
1 Grapefruit	EMI = 27.3

LUNCH

1 Baked Potato	EMI = 9.6
1 C Steamed Broccoli	EMI = 17.1
1/2 C Steamed Carrots	EMI = 13.0
1/2 C Steamed Zucchini	EMI = 32.1
Dijon Sauce	
1 Apple	EMI = 9.4

DINNER

2 C Brown Rice	EMI = 4.6
1 C Steamed Kale	EMI = 10.3
Tofu dressing	EMI = 7.4
1 C Squash	EMI = 28.8
1 C Savory Beans	EMI = 5.2
1 Pear	EMI = 8.9

Notice that all the foods are higher than 4.1 in EMI value. This type of diet can be eaten until you are full and you will still lose weight. Of course, you want to vary your diet from day to day, and if you do so based on the principles of the Eat More Diet, you will have a delicious diet that is good for you. The amounts will vary depending on your size and condition and the amount of exercise you engage in. Also, if you have health problems or are on medication, remember always to consult your physician before trying any diet. Individual needs do vary. For most of you, however, this is a way of eating that will support your good health for a lifetime.

PART II

How to Do It

CHAPTER 8

Getting Started

*A JOURNEY OF A THOUSAND MILES
BEGINS WITH A SINGLE STEP*

I've always liked Holden Caulfield's words at the beginning of the once-cult novel, CATCHER IN THE RYE: "To begin at the beginning, I began."

That's exactly what you're going to do here, you're going to begin. So—here's how the diet works.

FIRST OF ALL—Refer back to the certificate of value you signed in the first chapter. Remember, YOU'RE A VERY IMPORTANT PERSON! This book has information that will help you take care of that very important person. Now it's time to put the formula into action by following the simple steps you'll learn next.

GET EXCITED!

Starting now, GOOD THINGS ARE ABOUT TO HAPPEN TO YOU! If you follow the program, your excess weight will come off automatically and in all likelihood, you'll be healthier than you ever thought possible.

One of the best things about my practice is the joy I get out of seeing people become happy, healthy individuals because of the Eat More Diet. For example, Kathy was a 48-year-old nurse who went on the Eat More Diet. When I saw her shortly after she'd lost all the weight she wanted, she beamed at me. "I can't believe how my life has changed. I never thought I could feel so good, and it's been like this day after day. It's like I've been given a new life!"

So—get excited. This program can change your life in ways you never thought possible.

SET YOUR GOAL

By now you've reaffirmed what you want and you've reconsidered how the Eat More Diet can help you get it. Next you should set a goal: namely, how much weight do you really want to lose? 15 pounds, 20 pounds, 40 pounds, 100? Losing weight is made easier by setting goals. The following is a table you might use to help you set your goal. As you can see, there is a fairly wide range of what weight may be reasonable for you. The ideal weight for you will depend on many factors such as the following:

- Your build (The smaller your frame, the lower your ideal weight).
- How much muscle you have compared to the amount of fat on your body.
- Your age (The younger you are the lighter you should be.)
- Your race (These figures are based on studies done on Caucasians. Asians tend to be lighter, blacks and Pacific islanders somewhat heavier).
- Your health (If you have health problems) or risks for such diseases as heart disease, diabetes, or other obesity-related diseases, it may be wise for you to stay on the lower side of the scale.

Remember that there is constantly some debate going on about what your precise "ideal weight" should be. In any case, we know that most of America is too fat and we need to be more "trim." These tables have been set based on the recommendations of a number of studies that related weight to health and disease. (1, 2, 3, 4, 5, 6) They represent and suggest an optimal weight range for the best health and the lowest health risk. But there is a better way to determine what your ideal weight should be.

IDEAL WEIGHT TABLE (in Pounds)

inches	WOMEN		Height	MEN		meters
58	90	113	4'10			1.47
59	93	117	4'11			1.5
60	96	121	5'0			1.52
61	99	125	5'1			1.55
62	103	129	5'2	109	134	1.57
63	106	133	5'3	113	139	1.6
64	109	137	5'4	116	143	1.63
65	113	142	5'5	120	148	1.65
66	116	146	5'6	124	152	1.68
67	120	150	5'7	127	157	1.7
68	123	155	5'8	131	161	1.73
69	127	159	5'9	135	166	1.75
70	131	164	5'10	139	171	1.78
71	135	169	5'11	143	176	1.8
72	138	174	6'0	147	181	1.83
73	142	179	6'1	151	186	1.85
74			6'2	155	191	1.88
75			6'3	60	196	1.91
76			6'4	164	202	1.93

Estimates of "ideal weight" in pounds based on calculation of desireable body mass index weight (in Kg) divided by height (in meters) squared.

IT'S NOT THE WEIGHT—IT'S THE FAT

What's even more important than the weight is the fat in your diet. Many people weigh more than their "ideal" but are in reality quite fit. For example, many people who engage in body building might be substantially over the "ideal" weight in a weight chart but are in reality in good shape because their excess weight is in the form of muscle. The difference is in the body fat. When we talk about wanting "weight loss," we really mean "fat loss" which is desirable. We use weight because it is a convenient way to measure our progress, and we assume that most of the weight we lose is fat.

A better (but less convenient) way to estimate your personal ideal weight is to determine your body fat percentage. At the 1992 National Institutes of Health (NIH) conference on "Methods for Voluntary Weight Loss and Control," it was reported that there is wide variation as to what is the optimal body fat composition depending on age, build, and race. A good target is a percentage would be for men being no more than 15% in body fat composition and women no more than 22% in body fat composition with adjustments for the above factors. You can determine your personal "ideal weight" by having your body fat analyzed and your ideal weight calculated. Let's use two examples to demonstrate how this is done.

Example 1. Calculation of your "ideal weight" for a 150 lb woman

Let's take an example of a woman who is 150 pounds and has her body fat determined to be 35%. This means her lean body percentage is 65% and her lean body weight is 150 lb x 65% or 97.5 lb. In order for her to be at 22% body fat, you can calculate this by dividing the lean body weight by (100% - 22%) or 78%. In order to calculate the ideal weight, divide the lean body weight by the ideal percentage and you arrive at the ideal weight. Thus, 97.5 lb /.78 is 125 pounds.

In summary, to determine the maximum ideal weight of a woman at 150 lb starting weight, and body fat at 35%. (ideal is at 22%)

Current weight:		150 lb
Body fat percent:		35%
Lean body percent:	(100% - 35%) =	65%
Lean body weight:	(65% x 150) =	97.5 lb
Ideal max weight:	97.5 / 0.78 =	125 lb
Fat loss required:	150 - 125 =	25 lb

Example 2. Calculation of your "ideal weight" for a 200 lb man

Let's take an example of a man who is 200 pounds and has his body fat determined to be 25%. This means his lean body percentage is 75% and his lean body weight is 200 lb x 75% or 150 lb. In order for him to be at 15% body fat, you can calculate this by dividing the lean body weight by (100% - 15%) or 85%. Thus, 150 lb /.85 is 176.4 pounds.

In summary, to determine the maximum ideal weight of a man at 200 lb starting weight, and body fat at 25% (ideal is at 15%)

Current weight:		200 lb
Body fat percent:	25%	
Lean body percent:	(100% - 25%) =	75%
Lean body weight:	(75% x 200) =	150 lb
Ideal max weight:	150 / 0.85 =	176 lb
Fat loss required:	200 - 176 =	24 lb

GETTING YOUR BODY FAT ANALYZED

The down side of using the body fat method of calculating your ideal weight is that the means of estimating body fat are not as accurate as we would all like. There are four common methods of analyzing body fat, and while the field is constantly coming up with new ways of doing this, let me just say that there are inaccuracies in all four methods.

1. The "gold standard" has always been the immersion method in which the client is totally immersed in water and the water displacement is measured against her or his total weight. The problem with this approach is that the amount of air or gas in the intestines and lungs can throw off the results. Another problem is that it requires a pool of water and other equipment and immersion is difficult for some people.

2. The next most common method is an estimate using calipers and measuring skinfolds. The problem with this approach is that the technician must be well trained and results are very much subject to human error.

3. A newer method is electrical impedance measuring which involves using a device which measures the impedance of the body to a tiny imperceptible electrical current. It is a clean and simple technique which requires little training or experience.

4. Another new method is the infrared beam used on the biceps muscle. This is also a very simple technique.

All these techniques have reported about a 3% to 4% error for different reasons, with the immersion method being the most reliable but the most inconvenient.

Despite these inaccuracies, body fat analysis is a valuable tool in motivating you to lose weight and be at your optimal level of body fat. Just remember that there is always a possibility of some error and variation and use the results accordingly.

KEEP SETTING GOALS

Now that you know what a good target is, pick a goal that you believe you can reach. If possible, it should be within the suggested "ideal" range. Your belief and commitment is important to your success in losing weight. If you think that it is too hard to reach your goal in one big "bite" (pun intended), then set an intermediate or a short—ranged goal and do it in little bites. Set one that is more immediate and achievable such as a one-month goal, e.g., "I will lose ten pounds this month."

Then after you do this, continue to set reasonable goals. Be kind to yourself. No one reaches all their goals right on schedule so don't "beat yourself up" if you don't reach your goals exactly on schedule. If you don't quite reach one goal, set another. It's important to keep your ultimate goal in mind. Picture your slim, healthy self as much as possible even if you're not exactly on target each time.

Why does this work? Let me give you an example. When a plane leaves Los Angeles for Hawaii, the pilot sets the course of the plane. The ultimate goal and time is set. During the flight, however, the plane is almost NEVER exactly on course. It strays a few degrees or miles off course and the pilot makes some adjustments. It then strays off course again and the pilot readjusts the course perhaps dozens of times during the flight. It is probably OFF course over 90% of the time! Yet the plane ALWAYS reaches its destination. Your goal setting may work the same way. Just be sure that you keep a clear vision of your ultimate self at your ultimate weight goal and make your intermediate goal adjustments. Remember how many planes reach their destinations while being off course 90% of the time. You just may reach your goals in the same way in spite of yourself.

Typically, people on this program will lose about ten pounds per month. Some have lost as much as thirty pounds in the first month. This will depend on a number of factors, including how much you weigh when you start, your individual biochemistry, how closely you follow the program, and how much you exercise, i.e., have fun!

BE CREATIVE WITH THE EMI

Those of you who are skilled cooks may want to add more complex dishes than the ones provided. Pick your favorite spices. Use your own creative flair to spice the foods and garnish them and serve them in a way that makes you feel special. Make them taste and look good, for plain, sparse food often contributes to the feeling of deprivation that people get when 'dieting.' Below, you'll find a list of recepies that are meant to be a starting point. Use your favorite spices to customize the diet to your taste. One of the best parts of the Eat More Diet is the infinite variety of food it provides. So if you want to remake the recipes or invent your own, feel free to do this so long as you stick to the EMI as a guide when you're adding or substituting foods. And again, plan to eat more than you were eating in the past. Most people do at first, even if they lighten up later. This is partly because of the wonderful freedom you'll feel with regard to food that has kept you prisoner as you perceived and used it wrongly.

Get ready, too, for some wonderful surprises when it's time to clean up after cooking. One amazing thing you'll find is that you'll need little or no soap to clean your dishes. This is because the "fit foods" contain so much less fat and grease. There will also be less grease on your counters, walls, and cabinets. You'll find that your drain won't clog with grease. In fact, think about that clogged up drain. When I give lectures on the Eat More Diet program, I point out that if you have clogged drains in your kitchen sink, you're in danger of having clogged arteries. The foodstuff that you've been pouring down your drain to stop it up is the same foodstuff you're pouring down your throat, and it's almost certainly clogging up your arteries! Not only will your drains be cleaner, but your insides will be cleaner too. Now—you can either jump directly to the fourteen day menu plan in the next chapter, and come back to the section as you want to, or you can keep reading. Whichever way you do it, it's time now for action!

LET'S GO SHOPPING!

You may be at the end of the week and therefore at the end of your budget, or you may be able to go out and spend a thousand dollars to change your life and safeguard your health. Whichever it is, please realize that if you don't already own all the items in the following list, you don't have to purchase them all at once. Especially the kitchen helpers. You may want to purchase the implements and the new ingredients you'll need for the recipes day by day or week by week, as you decide to prepare recipes that use them. Or—you may want to go out and get as much shopping done as possible right now. Do whatever fits your lifestyle. Realize, also, that these are preliminary expenses, that once you've stocked up on these staples, you'll save a substantial amount of money by sticking to the Eat More Diet, even if you're eating twice as much as before! Also, the big ticket items such as the food processor are optional. While it's absolutely wonderful to own one, maybe you'll want to wait till the savings in your grocery bill actually start to add up, and then you can purchase it out of your savings.

BUYING KITCHEN HELPERS

1. Pots and Pans: If you're still cooking with aluminum cookware or using aluminum utensils, consider replacing it with stainless steel, glass, stoneware or cast iron cookware. Aluminum cookware can leave aluminum residue in the food which is cooked in it. If replacing your cookware is hard to fit into your budget, buy one piece at a time.

2. Grater: This will be useful for slicing vegetables and otherwise preparing food. If you don't already own one, buy one made of stainless steel. Well under $10 anywhere.

3. Steamer: A stainless steel vegetable steamer will be essential in preparing your vegetables and other tasty dishes. You can purchase one for well under $20 anywhere in the United States.

4. Wok: This is a Chinese frying pan that is shaped like an inverted dome with a rounded bottom. This is a good way to limit the oil in your diet as you can stir-fry your vegetables while allowing any drippings to collect in the bottom of the wok away from the food.

5. Pressure Cooker: If at all possible, learn to use a stainless steel pressure cooker properly. This I recommend because pressure cooking provides a way to shorten cooking times dramatically as you will see in the recipes. It also helps to lock nutrition into your dishes.

6. Food Processor: This will help you deal with the large volume of vegetables you will be eating. It's also excellent for making your own baby foods and has a thousand other uses. $50 and up.

SELECTING AND SHOPPING FOR EAT MORE DIET FOOD

Here are some general shopping guidelines that might help you select foods that make you eat more and weigh less.

GRAINS

Start with whole grains and other starches. This is your main course. As I have said repeatedly in this book, grains and other starches have been the center of the diet of every major civilization throughout history. Whole grains are preferable because they are medium in EMI and contain more fiber, which will expand and make you feel full. In addition, starches increase the thermogenic (calorie-burning) effect of food and help to satisfy your carbohydrate craving. Therefore, whole grains should comprise 50 percent or more of your diet.

VEGETABLES

Fresh produce and spices are especially important in the Eat More Diet. If you look at the EMI chart, you'll see that all the very high EMI foods are vegetables. You should eat as much of these foods as you want because, calorie for calorie, they will satisfy your hunger better than other foods. Quality is also important. If possible, buy organic vegetables and fruits. If you can't, don't be overly concerned. The cholesterol in all animal foods, and the fats in many foods are far more dangerous than the pesticides that you might find on some produce.

Select a good variety of vegetables. Be adventuresome and taste different foods that you have never tried before. And don't be discouraged. No matter where you live, you'll be surprised at the variety of vegetables available to you, once you step beyond the conventional potatoes, tomatoes, corn and beans that you grew up with. Stay away from canned vegetables as much as possible. The best is fresh, then frozen; use canned only a last resort unless you're diligent enough to do your own canning and can control your own quality and ingredients.

FRUITS

The advice given above with regard to vegetables is also true for fruits. If you live in a city, chances are good that you'll have access to any and all of the fruits you'll find in the Eat More Diet recipes. If you live in a small town or the country, unless you're lucky enough to be in the middle of a fruit farming area, you'll probably have to learn to occasionally substitute one fruit for another. This is fine, so long as you remember to substitute similar fruits for each other. Otherwise, you may alter the recipe's taste. Scan the markets in your area and try to buy the freshest product possible. Also, try to select recipes that call for fruits that are grown close to or in your area and plan your menus around fruits that are in season. Many fruits and vegetables lose their nutritional value as they lose their freshness, and this will lessen their value as fuel for your sleek new body.

NON-DAIRY CALCIUM FOODS

In the chapter on "Balancing Your Diet with the EMI," there is a section which gives the rationale behind looking for non-dairy sources of calcium. There are actually some excellent ones that we are all familiar with. Generally, they are in the leafy green variety or the sea-vegetable category of foods. In addition, certain foods have calcium added to them in their preparation such as tofu, blackstrap molasses, and tortillas if lime (calcium carbonate) is used.

ANIMAL FOOD

Though the Eat More Diet is centered on grains and vegetables, it is not a vegetarian diet unless you want it to be. For the purposes of the 14-day plan, however, the menus are without any flesh food. The reason for this is that the foods that are highest in EMI—the ones that will satisfy and nourish you most—are vegetables, fruits and grains. Flesh foods are nearly all "Fat foods." I want you to really experience the full sensation that the fit foods will bring you. If you want to add flesh foods, start by selecting those that are highest in EMI such as shrimp or certain fish such as tuna (water packed). Just remember that if you do use flesh foods, you must use them sparingly because they all contain cholesterol including the shrimp and the tuna.

But if you've grown up eating meats at just about every meal and you find yourself really missing the texture and taste in your diet now, there's good news! Today most health food stores and even many supermarkets have endless varieties of vegetarian products that substitute for meat, all the way from tofu hot dogs that are indistinguishable from the real thing, to "grillers" and "veggieburgers" that are better than any hamburger patty you ever ate yet are still made totally from vegetables. There are wheat gluten products also known as "wheat meat" or "seitan" which is made from wheat protein that has the chewy texture of meat which is excellent in stews and sandwiches. There are tempeh patties that pass for pepper steak or hamburger steak, and `Fakin Bacon' that looks and tastes like real bacon and is excellent in BLT sandwiches or with your oatmeal in the morning. There are also vegetarian substitutes for chicken, and for chicken stock. Vegetarian food production has come a long way in this past decade, and this is to your advantage because almost all these products are higher in EMI, and lower in fat and cholesterol than the foods which they can replace.

There's virtually no meat product that you can't substitute something vegetarian for, without losing anything to taste even while you make a tremendous gain in health and a tremendous loss in weight. In many of the Eat More Diet recipes, you'll learn to make your own meat substitutes. And if you can't get these substitute meat items, ask your grocer to order them and try them. He'll be surprised at the market for them, since people have generally become more health conscious. He or she will have access to manufacturers who sell veggie 'meat' products and you may even discover some I've left out here.

DAIRY PRODUCTS

Notice that dairy foods are not commonly used in the 14-day program and only the skim milk variety is used. This is because most dairy foods are low in EMI. Notice also that liquid foods are not on the EMI because water content changes the EMI unrealistically. For a better understanding of this, turn to the FFF—the Fat Finder Formula in Chapter 4. This has been provided as a general health aid that helps you always determine the fat content of foods, even when you don't have the EMI at hand. As I explained in Chapter 4, 2 percent milk is actually 35 percent fat by calories. Beware! This is just one of the thousands of deceptive advertising practices that exist everywhere in the world of food marketing.

The FFF is designed to help you see right through every one of them, so you can stick to Eat More Diet and fill your body with foods that promote weight loss.   So if you must have milk, choose skim milk as a substitute for whole milk or two percent milk.   Remember that more healthful sources of calcium are your non-dairy calcium foods such as your green leafy vegetables and seaweed.   But if you're not getting enough of these foods, eating too much protein, or have some other concern about your calcium balance, I'd much rather that you take skim milk or even calcium supplements, which have none of the negative qualities of milk.

GENERAL TIPS

Here are some general tips on shopping.

1. Choose whole foods over processed foods. Remember, we were designed around whole foods and our hunger drive is satisfied after the right amount of the right kind of food is eaten. And remember that any processing or adding of sugar and or fat cheats you out of food that you could otherwise eat. As you can see from the EMI, eating one gram of butter deprives you—calorie wise— of eating about forty grams of cabbage or some other equally nutritional food. Also, choose whole grain over white refined starches. Again—I can't say it too often— eat fresh vegetable whenever possible. Also fresh fruits are far better than fruit juices, since in most instances whole fruits have more fiber and they aren't loaded with tons of fructose— sugar!

3. Forget oily, buttery and creamy dressings, sauces, and soups. They're very high in fat and the lowest in EMI.   Stay away from salad dressings (unless they are the no-fat variety) and mayonnaise. Salad dressings range from 85 to 100 percent fat. Butter is 99 percent fat and margarine is 100 percent fat.

4. Watch out for sugared cereals. When possible, make your own from whole grains like couscous, oats and cornmeal. Barring that, read the labels carefully. Today, cereals, especially, make a lot of promises on the labels that simply don't hold up to closer scrutiny. Look for shredded wheat, grapenuts, whole oats and non- sugared puffed cereals to name a few.

5. Read the labels even on so-called `lite' products. There's been a lot of debate lately on just what that label means. This is also true of other labels, such as `natural' wherein there is no hard-and-fast rule that offers any consistency whatever. Several governmental agencies are trying to standardize labeling on foods so they won't be misleading. But thus far, it's caveat emptor.

6. Check out some of the other stores in your community if you can't find the foods you want at your local supermarket. You may be surprised at the exotic variety and the bargains you can find.

LET'S START COOKING!

You can either go, now, to the beginning of the 14-Day Program, where each and every day's menu is spelled out for you for the entire two weeks of the program, or you can take out a pencil and piece of paper and go through the sections on breakfasts, lunches, dinners, desserts and snacks and design your own menus. All the foods you'll find therein are high in the EMI, which means each and every one is a 'fit' food.

But you'll want to spend some time familiarizing yourself with the EMI, even though the recipes are all spelled out for you. Remember, this is a program you're going to stay on for the rest of your life, so keep sampling new dishes and find thosethat you like and you'll never be bored. You'll want to learn from scratch just what is and what is not good for you, so you can indeed begin eating right, so you can not only lose the weight and replenish your health but can keep the weight off and stay healthy. Take a copy of the EMI with you to the supermarket, and TRY NOT TO BUY FOOD THAT IS LOW ON THE INDEX! (i.e. lower than 4.1). This, in addition to the fact that you'll be full most of the time, will help you keep from falling back into your old, bad eating habits.

Remember—you're a very important person. And this is something you have to do for yourself—no one can do it for you.

But if you stick with Eat More Diet and let your hunger mechanism work for you instead of against you, this new way of eating will be the best thing you've ever done for yourself in your entire life.   And if you're healthy—and happy with yourself—that's a gift you can give to those whom you love and who love you.   You can also help them learn to eat right and avoid six of the ten leading causes of death.   So—

Here's to your health, and Bon appetite!

CHAPTER 9

Summary of the Eat More Diet Program

PRINCIPLES OF THE EAT MORE DIET

1. To lose weight, fill your stomach, and fill it with foods that help you lose weight. Use a positive approach by using the Eat More Index (EMI) as a guide to choosing these foods.

2. Enjoy your food. Flavor your food to your liking with low or no-fat spices and herbs. Savor your food and chew it well. This will help you enjoy the flavors and textures of the food. (To see what I mean, taking a mouthful of food that you like, chew it a few times and swallow. Then take another mouthful, chew it 15 - 25 times and savor the textures and flavors and see which you enjoy more.) In addition to increasing your enjoyment, this added chewing will do a better job in satisfying your hunger.

3. For easy weight loss, keep your fat intake low. Remember that "you are what you eat" and that high fat-diets produce high-fat people. Low-fat diets produce low-fat people. Try to keep your fat intake at around 10% to 15% fat by calories. On a 2000 calorie diet, that's 22 to 33 grams of fat per day. Try to keep the fat calorie content in your individual foods in general to less that 10% and at least less than 20% of calories if possible. Use the EMI table or the "Fat Finder Formula" to help you determine the percent of fat calories in foods that are not so labeled.

4. Learn to lose weight in your sleep. Use the three techniques outlined in this book to keep the rate at which you burn calories (your metabolic rate) high even while you rest. The following three items describe these techniques.

5. Listen to your body and eat until you're satisfied. If you follow the Eat More Diet, it will be almost impossible for you to overeat, particularly if your foods are high in EMI. A common mistake in dieting is not eating enough, then feeling hungry and going on a binge. This also keeps your body from lowering the rate at which it burns calories.

6. Fuel your fat furnace by eating lots of complex carbohydrates (whole grains and other starchy foods). Studies have shown that a diet high in these kinds of foods help you by increasing the rate at which your body burns calories even while you sleep.

7. Play your fat away. Exercise at least four times per week for at least thirty minutes at a time. While you burn some calories this way, the most important effect of regular exercise is to help you burn calories while you are not exercising.

8. Whenever possible, eat in a relaxed manner. As you probably know when you eat on the run or in a stressful situation, there is less time for your hunger satisfaction mechanisms to work and you wind up eating more than usual. Eating in a sit-down setting allows your digestion to work properly and gives your body time to let your brain know that it is satisfied.

9. Share your way of eating with others. It's more fun to do things with friends. This helps to support your own way of eating in the long run.

PRINCIPLES OF FOOD CHOICES

WHAT TO DO

1. Use the EMI as a guide to food choices. Eat whole food such as whole brown rice, whole wheat bread, beans, apples, potatoes, carrots, broccoli, etc. There are many choices of such whole foods and they tend to be high EMI foods.

2. To make your new diet approach as taste-tempting as possible, eat a wide variety of mid-to-high EMI food. To help you do this, use the "Inverted Pyramid" described in this manual as a guide. The following is a summary of the guidelines.

3. Start by making the center of your diet a whole grain such as brown rice or some starchy food such as potatoes or noodles at each meal. Have from 7 to 12 servings of foods from this group. In this way you will be likely to eat roughly 50 percent or more whole grain or starchy foods.

4. Be sure to have roughly 4 to 6 servings of vegetables per day, and 2 to 4 servings from the fruit group. This amounts to 25 to 30 percent or more from the vegetables/fruit group.

5. Eat roughly 2 to 3 servings of non-dairy calcium - containing foods such as broccoli, kale, collard greens, seaweed, tofu, and blackstrap molasses. This amounts to about 10 to 12% of your food. Remember that if you don't get your calcium from these sources, then you should add to your calcium with non-fat dairy products or a calcium supplement.

6. Eat roughly 2 to 3 servings of non-cholesterol, low fat protein/iron-containing foods such as beans and legumes. This should amount to about 10 to 12 percent of your diet.

7. If you choose to eat other optional food, do not eat them on a daily basis and limit the amount of these foods when you do choose them. These foods include dairy sources of calcium, cholesterol/high fat sources of protein, fats, oils, and sugars.

About Vegetarianism

If you choose to eliminate the optional portion of the pyramid from your diet, you will have a strict vegetarian diet. I believe that a vegetarian, whole-food diet is an ideal diet, but only if you are motivated and do it carefully. A strict vegetarian diet has the great benefit of containing no cholesterol which already makes it superior to most diets in at least one very important aspect. (1) There are also moral, spiritual, and environmental reasons to adopt such a diet if such reasons move you. (2)

If you decide to try a strict vegetarian diet with no dairy or eggs (also known as a "vegan diet") for an extended period of time, be careful about the B12 in your diet, particularly if you are pregnant or nursing. Vitamin B12 is necessary for the health of the nervous system and the blood system. The daily requirement for B12 is extremely small and most of us have about a three-year supply on board so it is not easy to become B12 deficient. B12 is found in small amounts in some fermented foods such as miso. There is controversy surrounding whether or not this is an adequate amount. A B12 supplement of at least 5 micrograms per day is recommended if you are pregnant or nursing or if you are strictly vegetarian for over a year. Be especially careful with the diets of infants and small children as their nervous systems are developing and are in special need of B12.

About Fats and Oils

Fats and oils are the foods that most often wreck diets. These foods are so low on the EMI that they hardly fill your stomach. In addition, they also have a lot of calories, so you wind up getting a lot of calories but still having an empty stomach. Oil does have a pleasant aroma so you may want to use it from time to time, but use only very small amounts when and if you must use it.

About Salt

Salt and even soy sauce are OK to use in moderate amounts for flavoring. In fact, in the standard American diet salt or sodium containing products are not the main source of sodium. The biggest problem is all the hidden salt. The three notorious salt bandits are 1.) Baked goods, 2.) Animal food, and 3.) Canned goods. Sprinkling salt at the table is actually OK as long as you don't overdo it. Salt is an excellent condiment and the best kind is sea salt. So if you are following the EAT MORE DIET, you can have a little sea salt, or soy sauce and enjoy.

BREAKFAST IDEAS

Although there are some fancy recipes in this manual for breakfast dishes, most people want something convenient for breakfast. Simple and healthful things for breakfast that are medium to high in EMI are:

1. Cooked cereal: Such as whole oatmeal, cracked wheat, millet, brown rice. Garnish with raisins or other dried fruit.

2. Whole grain toast: Whole wheat bread, whole wheat bagels, whole wheat English muffins. Use a no-sugar-added fruit jam or preserve or applesauce for added flavor.

3. Fresh fruit: Choose fruit in season, preferably from your locality.

4. Packaged whole grain cereals: Be careful about how much sugar is in the cereal. Use fruit juice or low-fat soy milk instead of regular milk. If you must use milk, use skim milk.

5. Reheated leftovers of all types.

6. Remember that in Asia, some people eat a breakfast consisting of brown rice, miso soup and vegetables almost every day! (Just go easy on the high-sodium miso. Make it light, i.e., 1 tsp per cup of water.)

LUNCH SUGGESTIONS

Another meal that often requires convenience for many individuals is lunch. If you work, one of the first things you should purchase is a good container to keep your lunch fresh when you bring it to work. A large-mouthed thermos is good for hot leftovers and soups. You can eat:

1. Sandwiches using whole wheat bread or pita pockets with filling made from leftovers from the night before or other prepared fillings (see section on sandwich ideas below).

2. Reheated bean dishes and soups. Also, these and other entrees can be served over brown rice, pasta or whole wheat bread or toast.

3. Other reheated leftovers with whole grain rice or noodles.

4. Salad and no-oil dressing or vegetables and dip served with whole grain crackers or other starchy foods.

5. Whole grain such as brown rice wrapped in nori.

6. Baked potatoes or other starchy staples such as sweet potatoes or squash.

7. Steamed vegetables with or without a low-fat sauce or dip along with brown rice or other starchy staple.

8. Soups: either prepared, or low sodium, low oil canned soup, or instant soup.

"IMPRESS YOUR FRIENDS" LUNCH

Here's a recipe to impress your friends with the Eat More Diet. Bring for lunch two baked potatoes with salt & pepper, two ears of steamed corn on the cob a dish of steamed vegetables such as broccoli, carrots, zucchini, your favorite low-fat dip sauce such as Dijon soy dip sauce, and an apple. Easy Dijon Dip is made by mixing 3 tablespoons Soy Sauce (low sodium), 2 tablespoons Dijon mustard, 2 tablespoons lemon juice, and 1 crushed clove of garlic.

2 baked potatoes	232 cal	270 gm of food	0.3 gm fat
2 ears of corn	166 cal	144 gm of food	1.8 gm fat
1 apple	81 cal	138 gm of food	0.5 gm fat
1 cup broccoli	46 cal	155 gm of food	0.4 gm fat
1 cup steamed kale	41 cal	130 gm of food	0.5 gm fat
Dijon dip	7 cal	45 gm of food	0.4 gm fat
Total	**572 cal**	**882 gm of food**	**3.9 gm fat**
		1.9 lb of food	**6% fat**

When they ask you why you have so much food, you can tell them that you are on a diet and that you discovered that you weren't eating enough food. Tell them that you have to eat this entire amount of food for lunch and a larger amount for dinner on your new diet. Then tell them that this is fewer calories that a quarter pound hamburger with cheese (with no fries or drink). If they ask you what kind of diet you're on, let them know that your diet tells you how to Eat More and Weigh Less.

SANDWICH IDEAS

Sandwiches are great for those who are on the go and need something convenient they can eat quickly. Sandwiches allow for unlimited creativity. Simply vary the breads, the fillings and the seasonings.

Sandwich Breads

The best kind of bread is, of course, freshly cooked bread from freshly ground whole grain, and baked without added oils, dairy or eggs. If you have a grain grinder and a bread maker, this may be feasible. However, for most of you, this is not always practical. So the next best thing you can do is shop wisely and select whole grain breads which are made with no oil or very little oil. Don't try to substitute "brown" bread, because it may not be made of whole grain. If you cannot find such bread products, commercial varieties will do. Here are some other options:

- Whole Wheat Bread
- Whole Wheat Burger Rolls
- Whole Wheat Pita Bread
- Whole Wheat French Bread
- Whole Wheat Chapati
- Whole Wheat Bagels
- Whole Wheat English Muffins

Sandwich Fillings

Start with a bed of vegetables that you would put in any "deluxe" sandwich such as lettuce, sprouts, tomatoes, olives, etc.

1. Bean dips: Bean dips can be used as a sandwich filling. The hummus recipe is an excellent example. If you are in a hurry, you can even find pre-cooked, no-oil bean dips in a can at most health food stores.

2. Prepared Sandwich Fillings such as imitation turkey filling are helpful. Be careful, however, because some of them (e.g. vegetable "hot dogs") are still very high in fat and low in "EMI".

3. Mushroom or Bean Burgers: These are also prepared with sandwich fillings such as "garden burgers" or "tofu burgers".

4. Pizza Sandwich: Spread prepared tomato sauce on a slice of bread. Season with garlic powder and oregano. Add your choice of vegetables such as mushrooms and braised onion, zucchini, olives, etc. Place open-faced in toaster oven and heat.

5. Taco Sandwich: Lay lettuce sprouts and chopped tomatoes on a slice of whole wheat bread or chapati. Add cooked pinto or other bean or bean spread. Add sprouts and salsa. You may also add avocado, guacamole or tofu spread.

6. Tofu Sandwich
 • Plain Tofu
 • Spicy Tofu (tastes like fried chicken)

7. Tempeh Cutlet Sandwich: A soy product which is quite delicious and is lightly fermented so that it carries neither a "beany" flavor nor a fermented one.

8. Sloppy Jim Sandwich: A no-cholesterol alternative to Sloppy Joe. (see recipe section on bean dishes)

9. Vegetable Sandwich
 • Kale
 • Tomato
 • Cucumber
 • Mushrooms
 • Sprouts
 • Zucchini
 • Other vegetables of your choice

Sandwich Seasonings

 • Mustard
 • Ketchup
 • Prepared Pizza or Spaghetti Sauce
 • Salsa
 • Tofu Spread
 • Vegetable Spike

• Vinegar
• Seasonings of your choice

SUGGESTIONS FOR SNACKING

Everyone snacks. This is a natural tendency. You can use this to your advantage if you know what to snack on. Here are some examples that are medium to high in EMI:

1. Corn on the cob steamed and eaten as is. (Hawaii is fortunate in that there is very sweet corn that is delicious without any flavorings.)

2. Air-popped popcorn with a little salt. However, because salt doesn't stick well to air-popped popcorn, a favorite trick of mine is to mix the air popped popcorn with a small amount of crushed lightly salted corn chips or japanese rice crackers (also known as "mochi crunch" or "arare"). It helps to give the popcorn variety and lets you taste a little salt.

3. Rice cakes with no-sugar-added fruit preserves, bananas or applesauce.

4. Whole wheat toast with no-sugar-added fruit preserves, bananas or applesauce.

5. Sweet potato: Another delicious, very filling, high EMI snack. Just steam or boil until soft and leave in the fridge (keeps about 2 to 3 days refrigerated).

6. Potatoes (n): Slice thin and place on foil in the toaster oven and toast. Flip them over and toast again. Make sure they don't burn. Sprinkle with a little salt or butter buds or sauce or no-oil dressing.

7. Raw or steamed vegetables plain or with dip. Some good examples are broccoli, cauliflower, carrots, zucchini, and celery.

8. Fresh Fruit.

9. Pita bread or whole wheat chapati "chips" with dip. Since most chips are quite fatty (corn chips are around 52% fat and potato chips about 60% fat by calories), making your own is a simple alternative. Simply cut the pita bread or chapati into chip-sized pieces and place in your toaster oven. Watch them because they may burn if toasted too long. Then use a delicious bean dip or salsa for dipping.

10. Brown rice plain or with nori sprinkles. A favorite snack of the Japanese people is brown rice mixed with tea eaten with nori sprinkles or salted vegetables.

11. Try to avoid snacking on nuts regularly as they are low EMI foods and high in fat (most nuts are 70 to 80% fat).

DINNER SUGGESTIONS

1. Try to plan ahead so that dinner is a cooked meal and you can save shopping and cooking time.

2. Seriously consider getting a pressure cooker. It cuts the cooking time for beans and grains from 10 percent to 50 percent.

3. Simple dinners are often the best. Brown rice, vegetable stir-fry and tofu is one of my favorites.

4. You can save time by cooking extra food, especially those that are time-consuming so that you have leftovers for the next day or to be frozen for a later date.

5. Remember that whole grain or whole starch is at the center of the meal and should be roughly 50 percent or more of your diet. (You'll recall that vegetables make up roughly 25 percent of your diet; 10 to 15 percent is high EMI calcium-containing foods; and 10 to 15 percent should be high EMI protein/iron-containing and other varieties of foods.)

6. Don't forget that simple steamed vegetables (naturally high in EMI) are great to have around as snacks and as side dishes for dinner.

LOSE WEIGHT WHILE EATING OUT

Eating out is a fact of life for most people. Of course, lunches are usually best handled by bringing your own, and dinners are often best prepared at home. But when you can't do this, here are some practical suggestions. Call the restaurant ahead of time and see if they prepare foods in the way that you ask. Usually, small family restaurants are more likely to accommodate you, but you'll be pleasantly surprised at the flexibility of some of the larger restaurants as well. Look for restaurants with salad bars or ethnic restaurants which may have vegetarian selections or near-vegetarian selections.

1. Ask the restaurant if they will prepare no-oil or low-oil vegetable dishes. Avoid or minimize meat, poultry, or fish dishes. This is an easy way to avoid low EMI foods. If you eat any flesh, avoid those which are fried, or cooked in a heavy or creamy sauce. Select steamed, broiled, roasted, or grilled selections instead.

2. Avoid fried, cheesy, creamy and buttery foods. They are very high in fat and low on the EMI scale.

3. To add a delicious no cholesterol-low fat source of calcium to soups, one of the best tricks is to carry wakame (seaweed) flakes with you and toss it in while the soup is hot.

4. Avoid restaurant salad dressings. Remember that almost all salad dressings are 80 to 100% fat. Plan ahead and bring with you no-oil dressing if you go to a restaurant that has salads. (If you must have dressing, have it on the side. Never pour it on and just dip your fork for the flavor.)

5. Bring other flavorings such as salsa, mustard, low-sodium soy sauce, lemon juice, vinegar, horse-radish, and no-sugar-added fruit preserves.

American Restaurants:
Perhaps the easiest food to order in a regular restaurant is a steamed vegetable platter with potato, whole wheat bread or rice. You can liven it up with your own sauces if it isn't done up by the chef with his own no-oil ingredients. You can also

order a baked potato with low-fat toppings in many restaurants. Another favorite choice is a large "undressed" green salad or pasta salad and use your own no-oil dressing instead.

Salad Bars:
Even steak houses have salad bars now and you can have a feast just at the salad bar. Just be sure to stay away from their salad dressings and use your own no-oil dressing. Minimize the use of nuts, seeds, croutons, olives, avocado, and salads with mayonnaise. They are high in fat and low on the EMI scale. Choose the vegetarian soups and sauces and avoid the creamy ones. Try to select bulky foods such as baked potato and whole wheat bread. Then fill up on a variety of vegetables. Ask for "A-1" or other steak sauce as it is tasty on potatoes. Pick fruit for dessert.

Health Food Restaurants:
You are fortunate if you have such a restaurant in your vicinity. Just be careful what you order, because many of these restaurants use fatty cheeses on their foods. Choose those foods that are without cheese and oil if possible. Their vegetarian burgers are usually quite good and convenient.

Chinese Restaurants:
Chinese restaurants can be surprisingly accommodating if you find the right one. Some of them already have vegetarian sections on their menu. Just be sure to ask for foods that are cooked with no MSG, and no or little oil. I like to eat vegetable chop suey, noodles with mushrooms and vegetables, and tofu or mushrooms with vegetables. If you go to a northern Chinese or Sczechuan restaurant, one of my favorites is "mu shu" vegetables which is "mu shu" pork without the pork, eggs, and oil. It is a dish of assorted vegetables (mostly shredded cabbage) cooked with Chinese fungus, and wrapped in a thin flour tortilla-like covering with "hoi sin" or plum sauce.

Mexican Restaurants:
Mexican food can also be easily adapted to vegetarian ways. Just order the Spanish rice and bean tostadas (or other bean dishes) without the cheese or sour cream. But be aware that most places use animal lard in the refried beans. You might look for restaurants that use vegetable oil instead of lard.

Some places allow you to order a la carte tortillas, beans, rice, lettuce, guacamole, and salsa. Then you can make your dish exactly as you want it right at your table.

Italian Restaurants:
Italian restaurants usually serve a good mushroom marinara spaghetti (without meat) or a plain marinara spaghetti. Just avoid the fatty cheese. Try to get the bread before it's buttered and season it yourself with marinara or other spices. Choose a vegetarian soup and an "undressed salad" to fill you up.

Japanese Restaurants:
Cold soba noodles (zarusoba) is one of the best foods you can order at any restaurant. Other things that are pretty good are vegetable ramen or saimin, vegetable sukiyaki, chicken tofu without the chicken (just remember that the stock is usually chicken, pork or beef based), vegetable sushi, (the kind with cucumber or yellow pickled turnip) and sushi rice.

Thai Restaurants:
Thai restaurants often have vegetarian selections. "Summer rolls" are vegetables and shrimp (you can ask to not have the shrimp) wrapped in a soft rice tortilla. They are quite good, and unlike spring rolls, they are not fried. Many Thai restaurants also carry brown rice. Ordering is similar to the style of Chinese restaurants.

Submarine Sandwich:
At submarine sandwich counters, you can order a tomato sandwich with just tomatoes, greens, onions, sprouts, peppers, and mustard with black pepper. Order whole wheat bread where possible.

Fast Foods:
While I don't like to patronize fast food restaurants because almost all their food is high fat and low EMI, I can say that most now carry salads which are reasonably good. Just use your own no-oil dressing. If you must have a sandwich, pick a burger deluxe, ask them to hold the mayo, and remove the meat so you have a tomato and lettuce sandwich. If you follow these instructions, you may have to order more than one (i.e. eat more) because these measures make the 'burgers' quite low in calories.

EASY START MENU

Before you change your diet, be sure that you check with your physician if you have any health problems or are on medication to see if such a dietary change is appropriate for you.

This menu is for the busy person who has little time to prepare food. It is designed to get you off to an easy start on this program.   Ideally, all your foods should be fresh and whole but when it's not possible, this is a reasonable beginning.

Basic Principles

1. Use whole foods if possible.
2. Your main dish is a whole grain or starchy staple and they are unlimited.
3. Vegetables are also unlimited. Try to eat at least five servings a day including some leafy greens and sea vegetables for calcium and iron.
4. Eat foods in season grown in your locality if possible.
5. Keep oil to a minimum or, better yet, don't use it at all.
6. Chew your food well (25 to 50 times per mouthful).
7. Make time to eat so that you can do so in a calm, unhurried manner.

DAY 1

BREAKFAST

Oatmeal with Raisins

For simple oatmeal, you can cook regular oatmeal according to directions on box, but without the milk. Before cooking, add a handful of raisins, a Tbsp of blackstrap molasses, and 2 Tbsp of wheat germ for flavor.

Fruit of your Choice

LUNCH

2 Corn on the Cob

Peel the husks off the ears of corn. Remove any bad spots. Place enough water in bottom of a pan to immerse the corn. Bring to a boil, cover, and reduce flame to low setting. Cook for 3 to 5 minutes and turn ears a time or two to ensure even cooking. Remove from pan and serve to a platter. It's best to eat it plain. If you want some sauce on it, umeboshi (salted plum) paste makes a nice condiment to use on the corn instead of the usual butter or margarine. Just spread a very small amount of umeboshi paste on the corn and this makes the corn taste even sweeter. Umeboshi vinegar is also very tasty. Just remember that these condiments are high in salt.

Low Fat Canned Soup (e.g. Hain(r) brand) with added greens.

Fortunately, health food stores now carry low-fat or no-fat canned soups. All you have to do is heat and serve. These soups are preferable to dry soups because the vegetables are generally fresher. You can make your soup even better by adding more fresh or frozen vegetables.

Some tasty additions include par-boiled kale, shredded cabbage, frozen peas, corn, carrots, broccoli, cilantro, sliced mushrooms or any other high EMI vegetable you can think of. One convenient suggestion is to take wakame (seaweed) flakes with you and toss it in while the soup is hot. In a few minutes you have a delicious calcium-rich food in your soup. If you load up the soup with vegetables, you may need to pour it into a larger bowl.

DINNER

Long-Grain Brown Rice

If at all possible, you should learn to use a stainless steel pressure cooker for brown rice. It tastes much better and cooks much faster (see instructions below). Or you can use a regular pot or a rice cooker as follows:

Steam-cooked rice

Cook enough so that you can have some for tomorrow's lunch.
2 C long grain brown rice
4 C water
1 pinch sea salt

Gently wash rice until water rinses clear. Place in 2-quart pot
(stainless steel if possible). Pour water to cover rice. Add sea
salt. Cover, bring to a boil, reduce flame, simmer for 45 minutes to one hour. Remove from flame. Let sit for 10 minutes
before serving. (Do not uncover rice while cooking.)

Rice-Cooker Rice

If you use an automatic rice cooker, use two cups of water to
each cup of rice. Wash and rinse the rice, add the water and
turn on the cooker. Adjust the water to your liking.

Pressure-cooked rice

For pressure cooked brown rice use 3-1/2 cups of water. Wash
rice and soak 2 to 6 hours (it will take a little longer to cook if
not pre-soaked). Place rice and water into a pressure cooker
(stainless steel if possible). Add salt, cover lid as directed by
manufacturer of pressure cooker. Bring to pressure on high
heat then lower to low heat and cook for 35 to 40minutes. Let
pressure come down, then let stand for 5 to 10 minutes, stir and
serve.

Cashew Stir Fry

- 3 slender zucchini
- 3 medium carrots
- 2 stalks celery
- 1/2 med. head cabbage
- 1 large onion
- 1/4 C mushrooms
- 1 C pea pods
- 1 small can water chestnuts
- 1/4 C cashews or slivered almonds
- 3 to 4 Tbsp soy sauce
- 1/4 tsp sesame oil (if necessary)

Slice zucchini, carrots and celery diagonally into 1/4" to 1/2"
pieces. Chop cabbage and slice onion vertically into thin crescents. Slice mushrooms into thin pieces. In a large pan or
wok, (oiled if necessary) saute mushrooms and onions in a little water with a little soy sauce until translucent. in 1/2 cup of
water over medium heat till just tender. Do not overcook. Stir
continually. Add 2 tablespoon cornstarch that has been mixed
with 1/4 cup of cold water. Add three or 4 tablespoons of your
favorite soy sauce. Remove from heat and serve over cooked
brown rice.

Steamed Greens

- 2 large bunches greens of your choice. (collards,
  kale, mustard, daikon, or a combination of two.)
- water

Wash the greens thoroughly, and chop into bite-sized pieces.
Pour about 1-1/2 cups water into a pan, add the greens, cover,
and bring to a boil. Reduce flame and cook over low flame
until just tender but still bright green. Remove to serving dish
right away to retain bright green color. Use a dressing or
condiment of your choice to season such as lemon and soy
sauce, Dijon mustard, tofu dressing, or sesame salt.

DAY 2

BREAKFAST

Grapenuts Cereal

Apple juice or 1% or fat-free Soy Milk

Your choice of Fruit

LUNCH

Brown Rice *(from last night)*

Pocket Sandwich

1 Whole Wheat Pocket Pita Bread

Stir-fried vegetables *(from last night)*

Fresh greens *(e.g. lettuce and sprouts)*

Slice pita bread in half so you have two pocket bread pieces.
Add greens. Then stuff with stir-fried vegetables. Add mustard, soy sauce, or seasoning to taste.

DINNER

Tossed Greens with no-oil dressing

Spaghetti(n) and Tomato Sauce

1 pkg spaghetti noodles
(preferably whole wheat or spinach type)

2 C bottled prepared no-oil meatless spaghetti sauce

1 C fresh or canned mushrooms

Cook whole grain spaghetti according to directions on package. Drain and toss lightly. Heat the no-oil or low-oil spaghetti sauce from the health food store or the grocery store with the mushrooms in a saucepan. Season to taste with seasonings of your choice such as fresh parsley, oregano, basil, salt, soy sauce, onion powder or garlic powder. Serve over the pasta.

Steamed Kale

- 1 or 2 large bunches of kale
- Water

Wash kale leaves thoroughly and cut on the diagonal into bite-size pieces. Place about 1-1/2 cups water in pan, add the chopped greens, cover and bring to a boil. Reduce the flame and steam greens about 1 to 3 minutes until just tender but still bright green. Remove to a serving dish right away to retain bright green color. Serve with tofu dressing described in "Dressings" section.

Garlic Bread

Fruit of your choice

DAY 3

BREAKFAST

Whole Wheat Toast with Fruit Preserves

Use hearty whole wheat breads, not just "brown bread" because "brown breads" may have color but not much fiber. If you can find bread made without oil, all the better. The fruit preserves should be made with no added sugar.

Fruit of Your Choice

LUNCH

Lentil Soup

Kale Sandwich

- 3 large kale leaves
- 1/2 tsp low sodium soy sauce
- Garlic powder
- 1 Tbsp lemon juice
- Whole wheat pita bread
- Dijon Mustard

Steam kale for two minutes and place in a small bowl. Mix the lemon and soy sauce and sprinkle some garlic powder to taste. Sprinkle over kale and chill. Slice pita bread into pockets and spread mustard. Stuff with kale and other vegetables to your liking and enjoy.

DINNER

Brown Rice

Seasoned Tofu

- 1 block firm tofu
- 1/3 C nutritritional yeast
- 1 tsp Spike seasoning (available at health food stores)

- 1/2 tsp black pepper
- 1-1/2 Tbsp soy sauce or tamari
- 1/4 tsp oil (e.g. olive or sesame oil) or spray oil such as PAM

Slice or break tofu into approximately 3/4" cubes. Coat non-stick pan with oil and heat at medium-high. Add tofu cubes and brown. Turn heat to low and drizzle soy sauce on each piece of tofu. Add yeast, spike, and pepper and toss, coating the pieces of tofu evenly.

Steamed Sweet Potato or Yams

- Sweet potatoes or yams
- Water

Place in steamer with 1" water and steam for approximately 30 minutes or more (depending on size) until fork tender. Slice and serve.

Steamed Collard Greens

- 2 large bunches collard greens
- water

Wash the collard leaves thoroughly, and slice on the diagonal into bite-sized pieces. Place in 1-1/2 inches of water and cover pan and bring to a boil. Reduce flame and steam for 5 to 10 minutes or just until tender but still bright green. Remove from flame right away and serve to retain bright green color.

Fruit of your choice

DAY 4

BREAKFAST

Brown Rice

Quick Miso Soup

- Wakame flakes
- Shiitake mushrooms, 4 pcs crumbled (optional)
- 4 C water
- Miso

Boil water. Measure 2 Tbsp miso (or to taste) into a cup and add a small amount of the water. Make a puree of the miso. Add this back to the soup and add wakame flakes and crumbled shiitake mushroom pieces. Simmer for about 2 minutes. Garnish with scallions or add other vegetables as desired.

Instant miso soup

If you must use an instant miso soup mix, add mushrooms, wakame flakes and other vegetables to taste.

LUNCH

Spicy Tofu Sandwich

- Spicy tofu (from last night)
- Whole wheat bread, pita bread or burger rolls.
- Vegetables of your choice such as lettuce,
    sprouts etc.
- Mustard, ketchup or other seasonings of your choice.

Use tofu pieces from last night and place in whole wheat burger rolls or pita bread. Add vegetables, season as you would your sandwich of choice.

Fruit of your choice

DINNER

Buckwheat Noodle Toss

- 1 pkg. soba noodles
- 1 tbsp grated fresh ginger
- Water, to cover noodles
- Tamari soy sauce, or Soba Sauce to taste
  (found in oriental section of markets or health
  food stores)
- Any leftover vegetables or beans, especially broccoli,
  peas, beans, beets (with their greens), cabbage,
  collards, dandelion greens, kale, mustard greens,
  spinach, turnip greens, all of which have high
  calcium contents.

Cook noodles in water according to package directions. If noodles already contain salt, do not salt cooking water. If they do not contain salt, a pinch of sea salt can be added to the cooking water. After the noodles are cooked, drain and rinse in cool water and drain again. In large bowl or pan, combine noodles, grated fresh ginger, and small amount of Tamari. Then cut lightly cooked vegetables (anything you choose to use) into bite-size pieces. Toss together with soba, warm—if you desire—and serve.

Wakame with Carrots (or other vegetables)

- 1/2 oz dried wakame
- 2 C large chunks of carrots (or other vegetables such
  as cauliflower, turnips, daikon, celery burdock
  or lotus root).
- 2 - 3 tsp low-sodium soy sauce
- (Optional) Scallions or parsley sprigs for garnish.

Rinse and soak wakame in warm water for 5 minutes until soft. Slice into large pieces. Put the carrots (or other vegetables) in a pot, and add water to half cover the carrots. Bring to a boil, cover and reduce the heat to low. Simmer until the carrots are nearly done (about 20 - 30 minutes. adjust cooking time for other vegetables). Then add the wakame and low-sodium soy sauce to taste and simmer until carrots are done. Garnish.

Tossed Greens with no-oil Dressing

Fruit of your choice

DAY 5

BREAKFAST

2 Fruit

Toasted Bagel with Fruit preserve.

LUNCH

Sloppy Jim (n)

- 2 C cooked beans (canned or pre-cooked beans such as pinto beans)
- 2/3 C tomatoes or prepared no-oil pasta sauce
- 1 onion, finely chopped
- 1/2 tsp garlic powder or 1 clove garlic, crushed
- 1 tsp soy sauce
- 1 tsp blackstrap molasses or barley malt
- Sea Salt

Saute the onion in water and the soy sauce until slightly translucent. Place all ingredients in blender and puree. Heat and spread on bread and top with lettuce, sprouts, and other greens, then sprinkle other condiments as desired.

Steamed Collard Greens With Carrots

- 1 large bunch collard greens
- 1 large carrot

Wash collard greens thoroughly and chop on the diagonal. Scrub carrot and cut into matchsticks. Place greens in 1/2 inch water in pot with carrots on top. Cover. Bring to a boil and then turn flame down and simmer for 3 to 5 minutes until greens are bright green. Serve.

DINNER

Tossed Greens with no-oil Dressing

Tasty Tacos (n)

- 1 pkg whole grain taco shells
- 1 bowl shredded lettuce
- 2 C chopped tomatoes
- 1 C chopped olives
- 1 C chopped onions
- 1 bowl low-fat refried beans (can be bought in
  most stores)

Slightly heat taco shells, fill with heated beans, then add other ingredients. Serve with salsa (can be bought in most natural foods stores) or make your own.

Salsa: fresh tomatoes, garlic, onion, cilantro, chile pepper, sliced tomatoes, salt, liquid from tomatoes,

Steamed Broccoli

DAY 6

BREAKFAST

Oatmeal with Raisins (see day 1 recipe)

LUNCH

Easy Pizza (n)

- Whole wheat pita bread (or whole wheat
        English muffins)
- No-oil or low-oil pizza sauce (from the bottle) or a
        No-Nightshade Tomato sauce.
- Mushrooms
- Zucchini slices
- Broccoli & Cauliflower cut into small pieces
- Other toppings to taste.
        Soy cheese is a no-cholesterol alternative
        to cheese. Use sparingly because of the
        high fat content and low EMI of soy cheese.

Spread sauce on whole wheat pita bread, english muffin, or
pre-made pizza crust. Add toppings. Heat in toaster oven 1 to
2 times as toast.

Tossed Greens with no-oil dressing

DINNER

Rice and Mushrooms

- 2 C brown rice
- 1/2 C fresh or canned mushrooms or 4 to 5 dried
        shiitake mushrooms (or a combination)
- Pinch sea salt per C of grain
- Soy sauce or Tamari
- Water

Rinse brown rice. If using dried mushrooms, soak mushrooms
in 1/4 to 1/2cup of water until soft. Reserve soaking water.
Slice mushrooms into thin slices. Add to rice and cook rice as
if cooking brown rice (described in day 1).

Steamed Cabbage

- 1/2 head cabbage, shredded
- water
- pinch sea salt

In a pan place water, sea salt, and cabbage. Cover and bring to a boil. Reduce the flame and simmer for 5 to 7 minutes or so or just until tender but still bright green. The sea salt will bring out the sweetness. Remove to a serving dish. For variety, you may serve with tofu dressing described in "Dressings" section.

Steamed Kabocha Squash
(acorn squash may be used)

Scrub squash clean, cut in half, remove the seeds, then slice into quarters. Place in pot (in a steamer basket, if desired) in which 1-1/2 inches of water has been placed. Cover and slowly cook for about 20 to 30 minutes or until it tests tender with a toothpick. Remove to a serving dish.

Wakame Vinaigrette

- 1 oz Wakame
- 1/2 to 1 C Sliced cucumbers, julienned carrots, sliced radish or daikon or any combination)
- Sushi vinegar to taste (available in oriental food section) or use brown rice vinegar mixed with a sweetener such as barley malt and a little sea salt to taste.

Rinse and soak the wakame in water. Thinly slice or julienne the cucumbers, carrots and/or any other vegetables. Mix with the sauce, let stand for 10 minutes so the flavor mixes with the vegetables. Serve as a cool, tangy side dish.

Fruit of your choice

DAY 7

BREAKFAST

Scrambled Tofu

Whole Wheat Toast with Fruit preserves

Fruit of your choice

LUNCH

Bean, Split Pea or Lentil Soup

Mushroom (or other non-meat) Burger

No-meat burgers are available in the freezer section of health food stores. Some of them are has mushrooms and tasty seasonings in them and is are available in some supermarkets and restaurants. They are convenient because they can simply be heated and served. Use them as you would any sandwich flavored with mustard or other garnishes that you like.

Baked Potato slices (n)

These are also easy to prepare. If you slice potatoes thin enough, for example 1/4" thick, they cook fairly quickly. In fact you can pop them in your toaster oven for 10 minutes at 400 degrees and put it through one cycle of the toaster and it will be ready. You can flavor them with salt and pepper or use some butter buds if you must.

DINNER

Brown Rice

Mu Shu Vegetables

This is a delicious dish that you can get in Sczechuan Chinese restaurants by ordering "mu shu pork" without the pork and eggs. "Mu shu" is actually a Chinese delicacy which is a crinkly dark brown or black fungus. This is difficult to find but not necessary to this dish. The secret is finding the Hoi sin sauce in the oriental section of a supermarket or in a Chinatown store. Hoi sin sauce is a savory plum sauce which can make simple vegetables into a feast. It is on the salty and sweet side so use carefully.

- Mung bean sprouts
- Won bok or head cabbage
- vertically sliced onions
- Mushrooms
- 1/2 carrot
- 1 clove garlic, crushed
- Hoi Sin sauce
- Chinese "mu shu" fungus (if you can find it)

If you wish you can also add
- cellophane noodles
- shredded cabbage

Slice cabbage and vertically slice onions into thin crescents. Chop mushrooms and cut carrots into matchsticks or grate it into thin strips. In a large frying pan or wok, saute onions in water and a dash of sesame oil until slightly translucent. Then saute the rest of the vegetables in water and soy sauce. Lay sauteed vegetables down the middle of a whole wheat chapati. Spread a half tsp of Hoy sin sauce on the chapati and roll the vegetables in the chapati.

Steamed Leafy Vegetables

MORE SAMPLE MENUS

DAY 1

BREAKFAST

>   *Oatmeal with Raisins*

LUNCH

>   *2 Corn on the Cob*

>   *Bean Burrito*

DINNER

>   *Long-Grain Brown Rice*

>   *Cashew Stir-Fry*

>   *Steamed Greens*

>   *Fruit of your choice*

DAY 2

BREAKFAST

>   *Grapefruit*

>   *WW English Muffins*

>   *Fruit Preserves*

LUNCH

>   *Bean Soup*

>   *Stir-Fry in Pita Sandwich*

>   *Green Salad with No-oil Dressing*

DINNER

Savory Lentils

Brown Rice

Steamed Broccoli

Spicy Oriental Topping

Fruit or Fruit Dessert

DAY 3

BREAKFAST

Brown Rice

Miso Soup w Wakame Flakes

Tea

LUNCH

Sloppy Jim Sandwich

Potato Soup

DINNER

Green Salad

Baked Potato

Mushroom Marinara Sauce

Steamed Kale

Whole Wheat Roll

Fruit

DAY 4

BREAKFAST

Whole Grain Cereal/Fruit Juice or 1% Soy milk

Whole Wheat Bagel

Fruit Preserves

LUNCH

Buckwheat Noodle Soup with Steamed Greens

Tofu with Ginger Sauce

Fruit or Fruit Dessert

DINNER

Tacos

Easy Spanish Rice

Tossed Greens

Fruit or Fruit Dessert

DAY 5

BREAKFAST

Oatmeal with Raisins

Apple

LUNCH

Burritos (using beans and condiments leftover from dinner)

Green Salad

DINNER

Mushroom Spaghetti

Tossed Greens

Garlic Bread

Fruit or Fruit Dessert

DAY 6

BREAKFAST

Kasha plain or with Soy milk

Grapefruit

LUNCH

Pasta Primavera

Whole Wheat Roll

Fruit of your choice

Steamed greens

DINNER

Bean, Pea or Lentil Soup

Vegetable Kabob

DAY 7

BREAKFAST

Cereal/Fruit Juice, Soy Milk or Skim Milk

Whole Wheat Toast

Fruit Preserves

LUNCH

Barley Soup

Brown Rice

Vegetable Kabob

DINNER

Easy Pizza

Salad with no-oil Dressing

Steamed Greens

Apple Crisp

*ABOUT NIGHTSHADE DISHES

(Nightshade containing recepies are indicated with the symbol (n)).

Nightshades are a family of plants which include tomatoes, potatoes, tobacco, eggplant, pepper. Belladonna, that infamous witch's potion, comes from the nightshade family. Some traditional cultures shunned this family of plants as food because of its reputation. Some of these nightshade plants are notorious for their toxins and are inedible, and even those that are edible can sometimes cause reactions in certain sensitive people. Even some edible nightshades have some toxins. For example, the eyes of potatoes may contain solanine poison, particularly when the eyes are sprouting.

If you're sensitive to nightshades, you should not use them at all when on the Eat More Diet. (Some of the symptoms of a sensitivity may be headaches, fatigue, weakness, indigestion, or arthritis.) However, not everyone has nightshade sensitivities, and for those who don't, nightshade dishes can be delicious!

SHOPPING LIST

For 2 Week Eat More, Weigh Less Menu Plan
(Actual amounts needed will vary depending on how much you eat)

Week One:

Starches

5 lbs. Brown Rice

Oatmeal
Wheat Germ
Pita Bread
Whole Wheat spaghetti
Bread (garlic)
1 pkg Soba noodles*
W.wheat english muffins
Taco shells
Chapati
   or whole wheat tortilla

Meat alternatives

2 blocks Tofu
Cashews/Almonds
Soy milk*
Miso*
Soy cheese**
Non-meat burger**

Dry Produce

Raisins
Lentils
Shitake mushrooms*

* Check the oriental section in
your store for these items
** You may need to go to a health
food store for these items

Fresh Produce

10 piece of fruit (various)

2 Corn on cob
3-4 pounds total:
  kale
  collards
  mustard greens
6-8 tomatoes
1 large pkg Carrots
4-5 Zucchini 3
1 stalkCelery
3-4 Onions
1 lb. Chinese Peas
1 head Lettuce
4 oz pkg. Sprouts
1 lb Mushrooms
1 clove Garlic
2 Sweet potato or yam
1 piece ginger
2 lbs. Broccoli
1-2 lbs Cauliflower
1-2 Kabocha/acorn
  squash
1/2 lb. radish or daikon
1-2 potatoes
1 head Won bok

Canned Goods

1 can Vegetable
  Soup
1 btle. Spaghetti sauce
1 can each beans:
  kidney beans
  garbanzo beans
  green/other type
   beans
pinto beans (16 oz)
1 can olives
1 can refried beans
1 can water
  chestnuts

Others

Wakame flakes
  (dry)*
Sea salt
Soy sauce (lite)*
Mustard
Garlic powder
Lemon juice
Olive oil or pam
No oil salad
  dressing
Salsa
Black strap
  molasses
No sugar fruit
  preserves
Plum or
  Hoy sin sauce*

Week Two:

Starches

Brown Rice
Oatmeal
Wheat Germ
Pita Bread
Whole Wheat spaghetti
Whole wheat roll/bread
1 pkg Soba noodles*
W.wheat english mufflns
Barley
Whole wheat tortilla
Whole wheat bagel
Taco shell
Whole grain dry cereal

Meat Alternatives

2 blocks Tofu
Cashews/Almonds
Soy milk*
Miso*
Soy cheese**

Dry Produce

Raisins
Lentils
Shitake mushrooms*

Fresh Produce

10 piece of fruit (various)
2 Corn on cob
3-4 pounds total:
  kale
  collards
  mustard greens
6-8 tomatoes
1 large pkg Carrots
4-5 Zucchini 3
1 stalk Celery
3-4 Onions
1 lb. Chinese Peas
1-2 heads Lettuce
4 oz pkg. Sprouts
1 lb Mushrooms
1 clove Garlic
2 piece ginger
1-2lbs. Broccoli
1-2 lbs Cauliflower
3-4 potatoes
1-2 Green peppers
Apples
Pineapple

Canned Goods

2 btls. Spaghetti sauce
Beans for soups:
  kidney beans
  garbanzo beans
  pinto beans
1 large can refried
  beans
1 can water
  chestnuts

Others

Wakame flakes
  (dry)*
Sea salt
Soy sauce (lite)*
Mustard
Garlic powder
Lemon juice
Olive oil or Pam
No oil salad
  dressing
Salsa
Blackstrap
  molasses
No sugar fruit
  preserves
Sticks for kabobs

* Check the oriental section in your store for these items
** You may need to go to a health food store for these items

CHAPTER 10

Eat More, Weigh Less
Diet Recipes

Basic Grains and Other Entrees

About Grains:

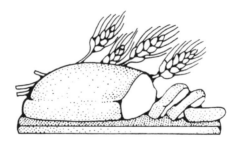

The top of the "Inverted Pyramid" is whole grain. It is the largest part of the pyramid and this should be the center of your Eat More Diet. This reflects the fact that the chief food of our ancestors and of people who have been slim for generations in all the great civilizations throughout history was a starchy staple, usually a whole grain product. In Asia where the largest proportion of humanity has lived, the chief food has always been rice. In Europe it was wheat and rye. In Egypt and down through the Fertile Crescent it was barley, millet and rice. In the Americas it was maize or corn. In Africa it was sorghum, wheat and millet. The ancient Egyptians even buried King Tut-Ankhamon (King Tut) with a cache of barley for his sacred journey in the after-life.   In some areas where grains were not available, a starchy (high complex carbohydrate) root was the staple such as taro in Hawaii. It is because of this central role in diets around the world that I recommend about 50% or more of the diet come from whole grains or other complex carbohydrates.

Rice is one of my favorite foods. It has been the principal food of more people in the world throughout history than any other. It is also the one grain that is commonly used in its whole form as food. Wheat, by contrast, is usually milled into flour and eaten as bread or pasta.

Whole Grain should be your main dish at your meals. I believe that one reason so few people cook grains is that there is some mystery involved in the cooking process. I hope this book helps to de-mystify it because we should be cooking and eating grains every day. It's actually quite simple once you become accustomed to it. As in cooking vegetables, pressure cooking helps to shorten the cooking time.

BROWN RICE

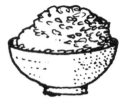

Brown Rice

- 2 C Brown Rice
- 3 1/2 to 4 C water
- 2 pinches sea salt

Steam-cooked rice

Gently wash rice until water rinses clear. If you have time, soak for 2 to 6 hours. Place in 2-quart pot (stainless steel if possible). Pour water to cover rice. Add sea salt. Cover, bring to a boil, reduce flame, simmer for 45 minutes to one hour. Remove from flame. Let sit for 10 minutes before serving. (Do not uncover rice while cooking.)

Rice-Cooker Rice

If you use an automatic rice cooker, use two cups of water to each cup of rice. Wash and rinse the rice, add the water and turn on the cooker. Adjust the water to your liking.

Pressure-cooked rice

For pressure-cooked brown rice, use 3-1/2 cups of water. Wash rice and soak 2 to 6 hours (it will take a little longer to cook if not pre-soaked). Place rice and water into a pressure cooker (stainless steel if possible). Add salt, cover with lid as directed by manufacturer of pressure cooker. Bring to pressure on high heat then lower to low heat and cook for 35 to 45-minutes. Let pressure come down, then let stand for 5 to 10 minutes, stir and serve.

Rice is Nice

Brown Rice with Wild Rice

Cook same as above, but mix three parts brown rice to one part wild rice.

Brown Rice with Chestnuts

Add several handfuls of chestnuts to basic brown rice mixture, cook as above.

Brown Rice and Barley

Wash and mix three parts brown rice with one part barley. Cook as above except simmer it for 45 to 50 minutes and let it sit for 10 minutes before serving.

Brown Rice and Millet

Wash and mix three parts brown rice with one part millet. Cook as above, simmer for 45 minutes and let sit for 10 minutes before serving.

Rice and Mushrooms

- 2 C basmati brown rice
- 4 to 5 mushrooms (fresh or dried)
- Pinch sea salt per C of grain
- Approximately 1 Tbsp low sodium soy sauce
- 4 C Water (3-1/2 C for pressure cooker)

Rinse brown rice. If using dried mushrooms such as Japanese shiitake mushrooms, soak them in to 1/2 cup or more of water until soft. If you want to add some additional mushroom taste, reserve soaking water and use it to cook the rice. Slice mushrooms into thin slices and add to rice. Then add soy sauce and cook rice as described above in brown rice recipe. Stir the rice and let sit a few minutes. Add more soy sauce to taste if needed while stirring.

Brown Rice and Quinoa

- 1-3/4 C brown rice
- 1/4 C quinoa
- 1 pinch sea salt per C grain
- 3-1/2 C water

Rinse grains gently and be sure to rinse quinoa thoroughly to avoid a slightly bitter taste. Place the grains in a pot, add the water and the sea salt, cover and bring to a boil. Reduce the flame and simmer for 45 to 50 minutes. When cooked, remove from stove and let sit for 10 minutes before serving.

CORN

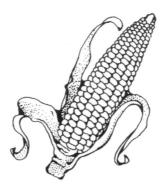

Too often, corn on the cob is forgotten as a grain and a main dish. Perhaps this is because it's too easy. What's even better is that it is the highest in EMI of all the grains. If you want to have something that is downright simple and delicious, try some plain, steamed corn on the cob. It is quite satisfying. If you want to spice it up a little, sprinkle some pepper, herb powder or butter buds.

Corn on the Cob

Peel the husks off the ears of corn. Place about 1-1/2 inches of water in bottom of a pan. Bring to boil, cover, and reduce flame to low setting. Cook for 3 to 5 minutes and turn ears a time or two to ensure even cooking. Remove from pan and serve to a platter. You can eat it plain or, as described above, sprinkle some spices on it. Make sure you stay away from using low EMI flavorings such as butter or margarine.

Easy Corn Polenta

• 2 C cornmeal
• 4 C water
• 2 tsp sea salt

Boil 3 C water. If you have time, for a slightly richer flavor, dry roast some of the cornmeal in a skillet until you smell a toasty aroma. Mix in 1 C water with the cornmeal to form a thick dough while smoothing out the lumps. Add the sea salt and slowly mix the dough into the boiling water. Turn heat to low, cover and simmer for 15 minutes. Pour into a lightly oiled shallow baking pan and bake at 375 degrees for 20 minutes.

MILLET

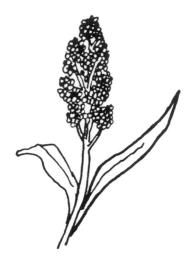

Millet is another grain that most people have never used, but it is great for variety. It can be used for a main grain with vegetables, it can be mixed with rice or some other grain, or it can be used as a breakfast grain. It can even be used with cauliflower to mimic mashed potatoes (see next recipe).

Cooked Millet

• 1 C millet
• 3 C water
• 1 pinch sea salt

Wash and rinse millet. Bring water to a boil. If you have time you can dry-roast the millet in a pan over medium heat until you get a toasty smell to bring out some of the flavor. Then place in the pot with the boiling water and add a pinch of sea salt. Bring to a boil and then turn the heat to low. Cover the pot and simmer for 25 to 30 minutes.

For pressure cooked millet, use 2-1/2 C water per cup of millet.

Millet "Mashed Potatoes"

For those of you who like the flavor of mashed potatoes but want to avoid nightshades, or if you just want some variety, here is an idea.

- 2 C millet
- 2 C chopped cauliflower
- 1/4 small onion minced (optional)
- 7 to 7-1/2 cups water
- Sea salt to taste

Wash and rinse millet. Dry roast lightly in a pan as in the millet recipe to bring out flavor if you have time. Place millet and cauliflower (and onion if you choose) in a pot with water, add four pinches of sea salt and simmer for 25 to 30 minutes. Mash the cooked product together or puree in a food processor while adding sea salt to taste. You may need to add some water for texture. If you are pressure cooking it, reduce your water to 6 cups and your cooking time to about 20 minutes.

Cooking Chart for Grains

1 CUP	REGULAR POT		PRESSURE COOKER	
	Cups Water	Time	Cups Water	Time
Rolled Oats	2-2.5	20-25 min		
Brown Rice	2	40-55 min	1.5-1.75	30-40 min
Buckwheat	2-2.5	2-2.5 hr		
Pearled Barley	2	25-30 min	1.25	15 min
Hulled Barley	2.5-3	1.5-1.75 hr	2.5	20-25 min
Bulgur Wheat	1.5-2	20 min		
Whole Wheat	2	1.5-2 hr	1.5	20-25 min
Oats, Rye	2			
Millet	2	25-35 min	1.5	15 min

BREAKFAST GRAINS

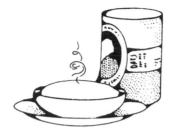

Breakfasts should be something to look forward to. Personally, I love the smell of oatmeal cooking in the morning. Breakfasts should also be simple. Some people enjoy eating just whole grain for breakfast. Some enjoy brown rice with miso soup for breakfast as millions of people in Asia do. Others enjoy just fruit in the morning. For many others who don't have time, instant cereals are all that are available.

Whatever you do, remember that it is most preferable to eat things that are prepared from fresh whole foods in season from your locality. (This helps ensure freshness.) That is, it is better to eat oats cooked from scratch rather than instant oats. It is better to eat brown rice than crispy rice cereal. But if you don't have the time, it is far better to eat instant or dry cereal than to eat bacon and eggs from a fast food restaurant. Eating such a high fat breakfast (usually over 50percent fat) is likely to sludge the capillaries in your brain and cause you to be less than optimal in your performance in whatever you do for most of the day. In addition, it is important that you eat in the morning because it gives you the energy to start your day.

Puffed Grain, Granola, or Whole Grain Cereal

Eat with fruit juice or low or non-fat soy milk.   Any of the
cereals can be found in a natural foods store and even in the
supermarket. Choose those with no sugar added such as shredded wheat; grape nuts; puffed rice, corn or wheat. Health food
brands such as Erewhon, Arrowhead, and Health Valley have
wheat flakes, bran flakes, or oat flakes to name a few that are
low in sugar. Watch out for some granola cereals which can be
very high in sugar and fat. If you've never eaten cereal with
apple juice, try it at least a few times. You may be pleasantly
surprised that it has a hint of apple pie flavor to it. Soy milk
can also be purchased in a natural foods store. Remember,
however, that soy milk has a fair amount of fat and that this
should not be done to excess.

Oatmeal with Raisins

For simple oatmeal, you can cook regular oatmeal according to
the directions on the box. Just leave out the milk if they suggest it. When the oatmeal is almost done, add a handful of
raisins. You may also add raw or toasted almonds or other nuts
sparingly if you wish. Just remember that nuts are low EMI
foods and are high in fat.

Raisin/Oatmeal From Scratch

• 1/2 C rolled oats
• 1-1/2 C water
• pinch sea salt
• 1/4 C raisins

Measure 1/2 cup rolled oats into a skillet, dry roast over medium flame, stirring constantly to prevent burning till the oats
are fragrant, a few minutes. Add 1 to 1-1/2cups of water and a
pinch sea salt. Reduce flame and simmer for 10 to 15 minutes,
until of desired consistency.

Cornmeal Cereal

- 4 C water
- 1 cup fine yellow cornmeal
- Fresh fruit to taste

Cook cornmeal according to instructions on side of box, or as follows if there are no instructions. Bring 3 cups of the water to a boil in a heavy saucepan. Mix the fourth cup with the cornmeal. Bring water to a boil, then add cornmeal-water mix. Stir constantly till cooked. If you wish, you can add a tablespoon of vanilla, or nutmeg and cinnamon to enhance flavor and to add variety. Serve the cereal with fresh fruit if you desire.

Kasha (Buckwheat)

This is a grain product that can be found in most natural food stores.

- 1 C buckwheat
- 2 C boiling water
- pinch of sea salt

Bring water to boil, add buckwheat, reduce flame and cook till soft (about 20 minutes). If you want to give the kasha extra flavor, before you add water, dry roast lightly over medium heat until it smells toasty. Then add the water, etc.

Breakfast Rice

- 2 C leftover brown rice
- 1/4 C raisins
- 1/2 tsp cinnamon
- 1 C water

In a pot or saucepan, bring water to a boil with raisins and cinnamon. Add leftover rice and simmer for 5 minutes.

Whole Oat Groats

- 1 C whole oats
- 5-6 C water
- 1/2 tsp sea salt

After washing the oats, dry roast them in a dry skillet until golden, stirring constantly to prevent burning. Pour water over the oats, add salt and bring to a boil. Cover and let simmer over a low flame for several hours or overnight. For pressure cooking, roast the groats as above, add water and sea salt, and pressure cook for 1-1/2 hours over a low flame after the pressure comes up. If made the night before, the groats can be left in pressure cooker and reheated in the morning.

FANCY BREAKFASTS

Sometimes it's fun to have a treat for breakfast. For those of you who want more than a simple grain for breakfast, try these dishes such as pancakes and waffles. There's even a scrambled tofu dish if you miss eggs once in a while. Just be aware that these foods are lower in EMI than whole grains and make it a little harder to lose weight. The scrambled tofu dish also has a fair amount of fat in it so use sparingly.

Whole wheat pancakes

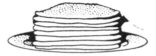

- 2 C whole wheat pastry flour or 1 C whole wheat pastry flour and 1 C whole wheat flour
- 2-1/2 tsp baking powder
- 1 Tbsp honey or other natural sweetener
- 2-1/4 C water
- Spices of your choice e.g., cinnamon, vanilla

Mix ingredients together gradually until smooth. Pour pancake size portions onto a non-stick griddle or pan. If this is not possible, use lecithin or a very small amount of oil. Cook until one side is browned, then flip with a flat spatula to brown the other side. Delicious with fruit topping.

Buckwheat Pancakes

- 1 C whole wheat pastry flour
- 1 C buckwheat flour
- 2-1/2 tsp baking powder
- 1 Tbsp honey or other natural sweetener
- 2-1/4 C water
- Spices of your choice, e.g., cinnamon, vanilla

Mix ingredients together gradually until smooth. Pour pancake size portions onto a non-stick surface or pan. If this is not possible, use lecithin or a very small amount of oil. Cook until one side is browned, then flip with a flat spatula to brown the other side. Delicious with fruit topping

Waffles

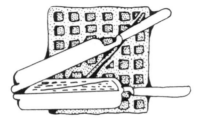

- 2 C quick or rolled oats
- 1 C Whole wheat pastry flour
- 1/2 C barley flour
- 1 Tbsp honey (or other sweetener)
- 3 C water

Blend ingredients until smooth. Let batter sit for 10 minutes. Very lightly oil and preheat waffle iron. Pour onto waffle iron. Brown, then serve with favorite topping.

Scrambled Tofu

Actually, this is not a grain dish but rather a soybean dish. I leave it in this section because it's a breakfast food that many find familiar in texture and appearance.

- 1 block tofu
- 1/4 C minced onions
- 2 tsp vegetarian chicken flavor seasoning
- 1/4 tsp sea salt
- 1/4 tsp onion powder
- 1/4 tsp garlic powder

Mash tofu. Saute onions in water while mixing in seasonings. Add tofu and mix thoroughly. Serve as a no-cholesterol egg substitute. (Note that tofu has a fair amount of fat.)

Healthy Muffins

(Contributed by Elaine French)

- 2 cups whole wheat pastry flour
- 2 tsp baking powder
- 1 tsp salt
- 1 tsp cinnamon
- 1/2 cup packed brown sugar, or 1/3 cup maple syrup
- 1 cup rolled oats
- 1 cup applesauce
- 1 cup fat-free soy milk
- 1 tsp vanilla
- 1/2 cup raisins

Preheat oven to 400 degrees. Lightly oil a non-stick muffin tin. Mix flour, baking powder, salt, cinnamon, sugar and oats in a large bowl. Mix applesauce, soy milk and vanilla (and maple syrup, if you are using it) in a smaller bowl. Add liquid ingredients to dry ones, add raisins and stir just until mixed. Spoon into muffin tin and bake for 30 minutes.

BREADS

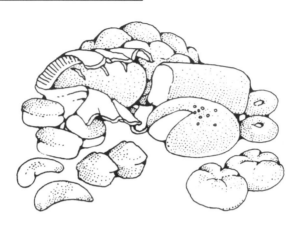

As in other flour products, breads are generally medium to low EMI and should therefore be eaten in moderation, unlike whole unmilled grain which can be eaten freely. This is because flour products tend to have little water in them and they are not as bulky as they would be in cooked whole grain form.

Simple Whole Wheat Bread

- 5 C whole wheat flour
- 2 C warm water
- 1 tsp sea salt
- 1 Tbsp baker's yeast

Mix ingredients together thoroughly, and let rise. If mixed well, kneading may be unnecessary. Place in floured bread pan and bake at 350 - 400 degrees for 20 - 30 minutes.

Pan Bread

Take a 2" ball of above dough and roll into a flat round shape. Then pan roast on a pre-heated no-stick or lightly oiled pan until lightly brown. Then flip and brown the other side.
For variety, you can be creative and add raisins, cinnamon, dried fruit, or vegetables such as onions or carrots.

Hearty Corn Bread

- 1 C corn meal
- 1 C whole wheat pastry flour
- 1 Tbsp baking powder
- pinch sea salt
- 1 -1/2 C water
- 1/2 C leftover cooked grain (optional for a different texture)

Dry roast the corn meal over medium flame until fragrant but not browned. Add whole wheat flour the last few minutes of dry roasting. Stir this mixture frequently so it won't burn. Let flour mixture cool. Warm the water. If you are adding the optional leftover, cooked grain, add it to the corn meal/flour mixture with your hands breaking up all the lumps. Add sea salt and the liquid in small amounts at a time until mixture is nice and thick but not too watery. Lightly oil an oblong baking dish and place corn bread mixture in pan and spread evenly in pan. Cover and bake in a 350° oven for 20 minutes. Remove cover and continue baking for 10 minutes or until golden brown. Allow to cool for 15 to 20 minutes before cutting into chunks and serving.

Garlic Bread

(Contributed by Elaine French)

- 1/3 cup fine corn flour
- 1 1/3 cups water, divided
- 2/3 cup boiling water
- 1/2 cup raw cashew pieces
- 2-4 garlic cloves
- 1 Tbsp yeast flakes
- 1 Tbsp dried minced onion
- 1 tsp. salt
- 4 tsp. lemon juice
- 1/2 cup sesame seeds
- 1/2 tsp. marjoram
- 1/2 tsp. dill weed
- 1 loaf whole wheat bread

In a double boiler (or non-stick saucepan) mix corn flour with 1/3 cup water until smooth. Gradually add the boiling water, stirring vigorously until blended. Bring to a boil, stirring constantly. Reduce heat to very low and cook for 5 minutes. Put corn flour mixture in a blender with remaining 1 cup water, cashews, garlic, yeast, onion, salt and lemon juice. Liquify until smooth, about two minutes. Briefly whiz in sesame seeds and herbs. Spread thickly on bread slices and broil until crusty and beginning to brown.

This recipe makes quite a large amount of spread. You may want to make just half a recipe, or to freeze half for another day.

ENTREES

<u>GRAIN MAIN DISHES</u>

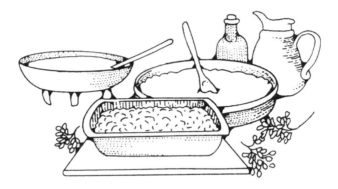

You can turn whole grains into an entree simply by spicing them up a bit and adding additional foods such as beans, mushrooms and sliced vegetables. Some examples of delicious taste enhancers are curry powder, miso, and powdered vegetarian "chicken" stock. Health food stores have many low-fat examples of packaged rice enhancers and helpers that can make it very easy for you to make a Spanish rice, an Indian curry rice, or some other delicious rice pilaf.

Basic Grains 'n' Beans

This is a basic rice and beans mixture. The trick is that some beans take longer to cook than the grain. It is simplest to use small beans such as azuki or lentils which take about the same time to cook as the grain. If you use larger beans such as garbanzos, soak them overnight and cook a little longer than you would other smaller beans.

- 1 2/3 C brown rice
- 1/3 C beans of your choice such as azuki or lentils
- 1/4 tsp sea salt
- 3 C water

Wash beans and rice until water drains clear. Add the 3 cups water and pressure cook with sea salt added for 45 minutes. Bring pressure down to normal and let sit in pressure cooker for 10 minutes before serving. Remove to serving bowl and serve.

Rice and Lentils

- 1 C regular or long-grain brown rice
- 1/2 C lentils
- 1 medium-sized onion, minced
- 2 tsp fresh ginger root, peeled and grated
- 1 garlic clove, crushed
- 1 Tbsp low-sodium soy sauce
- 1 tsp tumeric
- Boiling water (about 3 C)
- 1 large onion, sliced

Wash the rice and lentils together in water. If you have time, leave them to soak for an hour. Water-saute onions, ginger, garlic in fry pan, stirring occasionally until onions are translucent. Drain the rice and lentils thoroughly. Add them to the pan and saute gently, stirring constantly for 2 minutes. Add soy sauce and tumeric, mix lightly and cook for three minutes. Next, pour in enough boiling water to cover the rice and lentils by 3/4 inch. When water bubbles vigorously, cover pot, reduce heat to very low and cook for 35 to 40 minutes, or until the rice and lentils are cooked and all the water has been absorbed. Serve and garnish.

Sunshine Rice

- 2 C long-grain brown rice
- 4 C water
- 1 tsp tumeric
- 1/2 tsp cumin seeds
- 1/2 C green peas, for garnish (optional).

Wash the long grain rice and drain. If using a rice cooker, add rice and water first, then add the rest of the ingredients to the pot and turn the rice cooker on. The rice should be ready when the cooker automatically turns off. If using a regular pot, bring rice, water and seasonings to a boil, cover, turn on heat to low and let simmer for about 45 minutes. Add peas just before it's done. If you want "saffron" rice, substitute 1/2 tsp of the tumeric with 1/4 tsp saffron (a very expensive Indian condiment).

Spanish Rice (n)

(Courtesy JMT Miller.) (Cook a double portion, you'll use the leftovers in the next recipe, Cabbage Rolls.)
- 3 C brown rice
- 1 clove garlic
- 1 med. onion, chopped
- 2 C chopped tomatoes
- 1 Tbsp chopped pine nuts
- 1 bay leaf
- 1 small green pepper, chopped

Water saute (cover bottom of fry-pan with water instead of oil or butter) the onion, green pepper and garlic clove. Combine all ingredients in a sauce pan, add water till about 2 to 3 inches above rice, simmer 1 hour or till rice is fully cooked and fluffy. Serve with red and green jalapenos on the side, or may be garnished lightly with salsa.

Cabbage Rolls (n)
(Courtesy JMT Miller)

• 8-10 cabbage leaves
• Leftover Spanish Rice from last night

Heat rice, wash cabbage leaves, then stuff each cabbage leaf with the rice. Wrap leaf and fasten firmly with toothpick. Place on cookie sheet, top lightly with tomato sauce and one tablespoon salsa. You can also garnish with chopped onions and/or pine nuts (which may also be added to the Spanish Rice before stuffing cabbage). Bake at 350 degrees until tender.

Saucy Sandwich (n)

• 2 slices whole wheat bread, or 1 whole wheat chapati, tortilla, or pita bread
• 1/2 C broccoli
• 1/2 C cauliflower
• 1 C lettuce, shredded
• 1/2 C alfalfa sprouts
• 3 Tbsp carrots, grated
• 1/4 C sauteed onions
• 2 tsp no fat or tofu dressing (optional)

Onion Barbecue Sauce

• 1 small round onion, diced
• 1 Tbsp water
• 1 Tbsp barbecue sauce

Saute onions in water and oil until slightly translucent. Then add barbecue sauce and saute until soft. Use as a sauce for the sandwich. As an option you can add or substitute mushrooms.

Mushroom Teriyaki Sauce

- 1/2 C mushrooms
- 1 tsp arrowroot or cornstarch
- 2 Tbsp water
- 2 Tbsp low sodium soy or tamari
- 1 tsp molasses or honey
- 1 tsp grated ginger (optional)

Chop mushrooms into small pieces. Add soy sauce, honey and ginger and saute with mushrooms. Dissolve arrowroot in cool water and add to mushrooms. Add water for desired consistency and continue to saute for a minute or so until the ingredients are blended. Use on vegetables in sandwich, or use on beans, tofu, or mix with noodles.

PASTAS

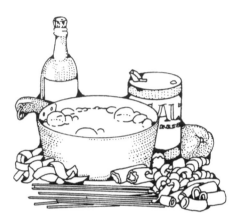

Pastas are another delicious staple food to help you lose weight. They are not as high in EMI as whole grains such as rice, corn and millet because, after all, pastas are made from flour. However, I like pastas because unlike many other flour products such as baked goods, pastas have no added oil. This tends to make them higher in EMI and satisfaction value than bread but not as high as an unmilled grain such as brown rice or millet. As in all flour products, it is better to get the whole grain type of pasta such as whole wheat noodles or buckwheat noodles rather than pasta made from refined flour.

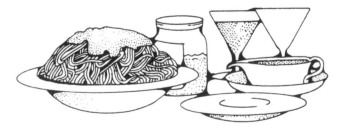

Basic Pasta

Most pastas have their own instructions for preparation printed on the package. One simple technique is to boil enough water to immerse the pasta in a pot, place the pasta in the boiling water, turn off the heat and cover the pot. About 10 to 15 minutes later, depending on the thickness of the pasta, it's ready. Buckwheat noodles (soba) need special attention because as it boils, it foams and will overflow unless you pour cool water in small amounts into the saucepan as it boils over. You'll have to do this about three times before it is cooked. Pastas can be eaten with any number of delicious sauces or side dishes. For some examples, see the section to follow on "Grain Main Dishes".

Spaghetti and Tomato Sauce (n)

Cook spaghetti (preferably whole grain) noodles according to directions on package or as described above. Drain and, if you wish, add chopped fresh parsley. Serve with tomato sauce:

Tomato Sauce

- 4 minced garlic cloves
- 4 C canned tomatoes with juice
- 1 C tomato paste
- 2 tsp basil
- 1 tsp oregano
- 1-3/4 tsp salt
- 1 Tbsp honey
- low sodium soy sauce
- Optional additional ingredients such as chopped mushrooms and/or broccoli flowerettes

In pot, saute garlic in water and a little soy sauce. Add onions and saute until soft. Add tomatoes, squashing with hands. Add remaining ingredients. Stir together. Simmer for one hour to blend flavors. Add soy sauce or salt to taste.

No-Nightshade Tomato Sauce

For those of you who want to avoid nightshades, here's a tomato sauce substitute. You'll be amazed at how much like tomato sauce it turns out to be.

- 5 C carrots (about 5 to 6)
- 2/3 C beets (about one beet)
  (adjust ratio of carrots to beets for color).
- 1 medium onion, chopped
- 1 bay leaf
- 3 garlic cloves, minced
- 1-1/2 C water
- 3 umeboshi plum - pitted (a tart Japanese salted plum found in health food stores or where Japanese foods are sold.)
- 1 tsp basil
- 1 tsp oregano
- low sodium soy sauce
- 1 C mushrooms

Place carrots, beets, onion, bay leaf, garlic, umeboshi and spices in a pot and boil for 30 minutes. Saute onion, garlic and mushrooms in water and a little soy sauce. Place all other ingredients in blender and blend. Then mix in onion, garlic and mushrooms with the blended ingredients. Add extras to tailor to your own family recipe as desired. Use this instead of tomato in pizza, spaghetti, tacos, etc.

Pasta Primavera

Pasta:

3/4 lb pasta of your choice (such as whole wheat or spinach fettucini, linguini, spiral pasta or your favorite pasta).

- 2 quarts (8 C) water
- Vegetables:
- 1 C broccoli flowerettes
- 1 C cauliflower flowerettes
- 1 carrot, sliced
- 1 zucchini, sliced

- 1-1/2 C mushrooms, sliced
- 2 cloves garlic, crushed
- 1 Tbsp low sodium soy sauce
- 1 tsp olive oil (optional)

Sauce:

- 1 C water
- 2/3 C soy milk (low fat preferred)
- 2 Tbsp arrowroot (or cornstarch)
- 1 Tbsp Dijon mustard
- 1 Tbsp low sodium soy sauce
- 1 tsp basil
- black pepper and other spices to taste.

Bring the 2 quarts water to boil. Place pasta in boiling water, turn off heat and cover the pot. Let stand for 12 - 15 minutes or until tender then drain. Place vegetables in a pan with water or a mixture of water and oil. Water saute the vegetables while adding soy sauce. Dissolve the arrowroot in small amount of water and then mix with soy sauce, water, and dijon in a saucepan. Add the basil while simmering at medium heat until desired texture is achieved. Combine the pasta, sauce, and vegetables and toss for a delicious pasta primavera.

Basic Buckwheat Noodles

Buckwheat noodles are one of my favorite pasta dishes because it is the one pasta made from whole grain that is commonly served even in restaurants. At Japanese restaurants, it is served hot or cold and is an excellent basic cereal grain product around which to plan a meal.

- 1 pkg. buckwheat (soba) noodle
- 1 Tbsp chopped green onion
- 1 can or bottle Japanese soba sauce or prepare dip sauce below
- (optional) nori flakes

Boil enough water to immerse the noodles in a pot, and place the noodles in the boiling water. As it boils, it will foam so before it overflows, pour a small amount of cool water into the saucepan and the foaming will stop for a short while and will build up again. You'll have to do this about three times before it is cooked. If noodles already contain salt, do not salt cooking water. If they do not contain salt, a pinch of sea salt can be added to the cooking water. After the noodles are cooked, drain and rinse in cool water and drain again. Garnish with green onion, and if you have them, nori flakes, and serve cold. Use the sauce for flavor as a dipping sauce.

Prepare dipping sauce using:

- 1/4C low-sodium soy sauce
  (for the simplest sauce you can just use soy sauce)
- 2 C water
- 1 piece of konbu about 3" x 2"
- 1 tsp grated ginger

Boil the konbu in water for 5 minutes and remove the konbu (it can be sliced and eaten with other vegetables). Then add the other ingredients. You can vary the taste of the sauce by optionally adding the ingredients below.

- 1 tsp wasabi (Japanese horseradish, the kind used on sushi)
- 1 to 2 tsp lemon juice for a tangy taste
- 1 crushed clove garlic

Serve in separate bowls for each person to dip their noodles.

Buckwheat Noodle Medley

- 1 pkg. buckwheat (soba) noodles
- 1 tbsp grated fresh ginger
- Water to cover noodles
- Water to cool noodles while cooking
- Low sodium soy sauce, to taste
- Any leftover vegetables or beans, especially broccoli, peas,
  beans, cabbage, collards, kale, mustard greens, spinach,
  turnip greens.

Prepare noodles as above. In large bowl or pan, combine noodles, grated fresh ginger, and small amount of low sodium soy sauce or tamari. Then cut lightly cooked vegetables *(anything you choose to use)* into bite-size pieces. Toss together with soba, cold or warm—if you desire—and serve.

Canneloni (n)

(contributed by Ann Tang)

This recipe is well worth the effort and is absolutely delicious.

Sauce:

- 3 cloves garlic, minced
- 1 round onion, chopped
- 6 fresh tomatoes, skinned and chopped
- 1 large can whole tomatoes, chopped
- 6 fresh basil leaves, chopped
- 1 tsp oregano
- 1 Tbsp cilantro
- 1 lb. fresh mushrooms, sliced
- 1/2 C red wine

Saute garlic and round onion in 1 cup water until transparent. Add fresh and canned tomatoes and simmer 30 minutes. Add rest of the ingredients and simmer another 30 minutes.

Optional: Season to taste with apple and lemon juice
         1/4 tsp red chili pepper flakes

Filling:

- 2 cloves garlic, minced
- 1 round onion, chopped
- 2 bunches fresh spinach, chopped
- 2 C fresh mushrooms, diced
- 1 C shiitake mushrooms, soaked in water and finely diced (optional)
- 1 C cooked organic barley
- 2 C firm tofu
- 1 C corn

Saute garlic and onion in 1 cup water until transparent. Add shiitake mushrooms and simmer 10 minutes to soften. Add remainder of ingredients and simmer 15 minutes.

Cool and fill uncooked cannelloni shells. Place in baking pan and top with any leftover filling. Pour sauce over stuffed shells and bake covered at 350°, 45-60 minutes. Bake uncovered last 15 minutes.

Preparation Time: 20-30 minutes
Cooking Time: 1-1/2-2 hours

Garlic Noodles

• 1 pkg. whole wheat noodles
• 2 to 3 medium cloves garlic (diced)
• Water

Try to select these noodles or pasta for variety. I like to use the broader flat noodle such as fettucine although any pasta will do. Cook noodles according to package directions. If noodles do not have salt in their ingredients, add 1/4 teaspoon of salt to the cooking water. While noodles cook, peel garlic and dice. When noodles are ready, drain into a colander and rinse with cool water, let drain. Saute garlic in a small amount of sesame oil. Add cooked noodles and toss with garlic, heat through and serve.

Pasta & Oriental Mushroom Gravy

Cook whole grain spaghetti or other pasta according to directions on package or as described above. Drain, garnish with either fresh chopped parsley, cilantro, or dried parsley and cilantro. Top with Oriental Mushroom Gravy

• 4 C water
• 6 Tbsp low sodium soy sauce or tamari
• 5 Tbsp cornstarch or arrowroot
• 1-1/2 C chopped fresh mushrooms or dried shiitake mushrooms
• optional Tbsp grated ginger

Dissolve cornstarch in cool water. Then mix in soy sauce, pour into saucepan and add mushrooms. Cook, stirring constantly, over medium-high heat until thickened. If using dried mushrooms, soak in water for a few minutes and slice mushrooms. You may save the soaking water to replace some of the water in this recipe for more mushroom flavor.

STIR FRYS

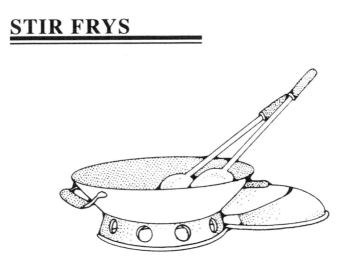

Stir frys are one of my favorites because they are easy, tasty and infinite in variety. They are also usually very high in EMI so they fill you right up. You can make them any way you want with any ingredients so be creative. It's easy to use foods that are high in EMI such as broccoli, mushrooms, carrots, onions, zucchini, and cabbage to name a few examples of ingredients. It is preferable to avoid oil. Try doing so by water saute and flavor the stir fry using low sodium soy sauce or tamari, herbs, spices, mustard, or any other condiments. If you want to thicken it, use arrowroot or corn starch. If you use oil, make it a small amount.

Cashew Stir Fry

- 3 slender zucchini
- 3 medium carrots
- 2 stalks celery
- 1/2 med. head cabbage or Chinese cabbage
- 1 large onion
- 1 C pea pods
- 1 small can water chestnuts
- 1/4 C cashews or slivered almonds
- 3 to 4 Tbsp soy sauce
- optional 1 tsp sesame oil

Slice the zucchini, carrots, and celery diagonally. Chop the cabbage and slice the onion vertically into crescents. If using oil, saute the onions lightly with oil first. Otherwise, saute in water and soy sauce. Then add other vegetables and cashews with 1/2 cup of water over medium heat till just tender. Do not overcook. Stir continually in wok or large frying pan while adding soy sauce. If you want to thicken the moisture in the stir-fry, add 2 tablespoon cornstarch that has been mixed with 1/2 cup of cold water and stir-fry for a few minutes. Remove from heat and serve with cooked brown rice.

Chinese Stir-Fry Supreme

- 1/2 lb tofu, cut in 1" squares
- 4 shiitake mushrooms
- 1 onion
- 3 stalks celery
- 2 C Chinese or regular cabbage finely cut
- 3 C mung bean sprouts
- 3 Tbsp arrowroot
- 3 Tbsp low-sodium soy sauce or tamari
- 1 tsp sesame oil (optional)

Slice onions vertically into crescents, chop celery diagonally into 1/2" pieces, chop cabbage, and soak and slice the mush-rooms. Brown tofu well on all sides on low heat in a non-stick skillet with oil until it slides around in the pan. Add mush-rooms and a little soy sauce and saute a little longer. Saute ·

onion, celery, cabbage, and sprouts in a large skillet or wok. Add enough water to cover. When it boils, add arrowroot dissolved in cool water to thicken. Let cook for 3 to 4 minutes. Add soy sauce to taste, mix in tofu and mushrooms and pour immediately into serving dish. Serve with buckwheat noodles, whole wheat noodles, or brown rice.

Mu Shu Vegetables

(See day 7 of menu)

KABOBS

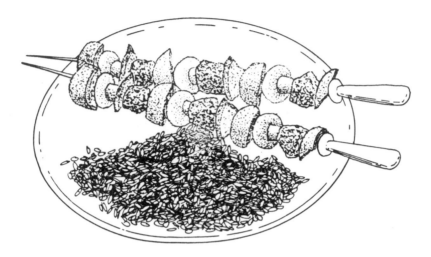

Kabobs can be a festive treat and relatively easy to prepare. They are also another way to use high EMI foods. I got interested in kabobs when a patient of mine said that she had to go to a potluck dinner where they were all making kabobs and didn't know what to bring. I told her she could easily bring delicious vegetable kabobs. The secret, I told her was in the marinade. The happy ending was that everyone liked her kabobs best and many of them wound up leaving the meat off their kabobs and borrowing her marinade.

Vegetable Kabobs

- 1 small cauliflower (flowerettes)
- 10 string beans or 1 bunch broccoli (flowerettes)
- 2 carrots cut into 1 inch pieces
- 3 stalks celery cut into 1 inch pieces
- 1/2 block firm tofu or tempeh (a soybean product fermented just enough to reduce some of the beany taste and gas) cut into cubes.
- Sea salt

Bring 2 to 3 inches of water to a boil and steam tofu or tempeh and vegetables until just tender. On a skewer place pieces of carrot, celery, string bean, and cauliflower. Place the cauliflower on the end so it will look like a flower on the end of the skewer. Top kabobs with sauce. As a variation, you can marinate the kabobs in the sauce and then cook over a grill.

Sauces for Kabobs

Dijon Marinade

- 2 Tbsp Dijon mustard (for variation, use other mustards)
- 3 Tbsp low-sodium soy sauce or tamari
- 3 Tbsp lemon juice
- 2 cloves garlic, crushed

Mix ingredients together and use as marinade.

Teriyaki Marinade

- 1/3 C low-sodium soy sauce or tamari
- 2 Tbsp blackstrap molasses or honey
- 1 Tbsp grated ginger
- 1 clove garlic crushed
- 2 tsp arrowroot or corn starch
- 2 Tbsp water
- 1 Tbsp sake or white wine (optional)
- 1 Tbsp lemon juice (optional)

Mix the arrowroot to dissolve in water. Then combine with other ingredients in a saucepan. Bring to a boil and let cool.

Korean Barbecue Sauce

Follow teriyaki marinade instructions but use 3 cloves garlic, no ginger, and add 1/2 tsp sesame oil.

White Wine Marinade

- 1/2 C white wine
- 2 Tbsp lemon juice
- 2 to 3 bay leaves
- 3/4 tsp thyme
- pepper

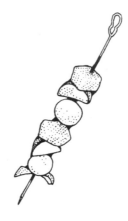

Mix ingredients together and it's ready.

Barbecue Marinade.

- 3/4 C ketchup
- 1/4 C lemon juice
- 3 Tbsp molasses or honey
- 1/4 C steak sauce (i.e. A-1 steak sauce)
- 1/2 tsp sea salt
- pepper

Mix ingredients and boil, cover and simmer for 4 - 5 minutes.

SAVORY BEAN DISHES

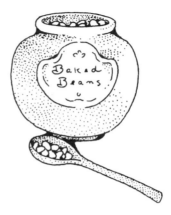

Bean dishes are delicious, hearty and filling. They are excellent weight loss dishes when prepared properly. They are moderate to high in EMI and provide an excellent protein source. They also make delicious spreads that are very low in fat (as long as you don't add any fats). If you don't have time to cook, you can get beans in a can at the supermarket or the health food store. I do advise you to rinse the beans because they can be salty due to the salt added to the can to retard spoilage.

Here is a simple bean suggestion if you are busy. Take a can of no-oil or no-fat refried beans. Heat it up and add 1 box frozen lima beans and 1 box frozen corn 1/2 red pepper, 1 crushed garlic. Simmer 20 to 30 min, add chili flakes and heat

Tips for Eliminating Gas: Beans can be gassy if they are not cooked properly or if you do not chew properly. Gas develops when undigested protein or starch get to the large intestine providing food for the flora that resides there. Here are some tips eliminate gas.

1. Soak overnight and pour off water.
2. Boil for ten minutes and pour off foam before cooking
3. Cook thoroughly (see table below)
4. Chew thoroughly.

Cooking Chart for Beans

1 CUP	Cups Water	Time	Water	Time
	REGULAR POT		**PRESSURE COOKER**	
Lentils	3	30-60 min	to cover	25-45 min
Split Peas	2-3	30-60 min	1/2"over	20-40 min
Black Beans	4	1.5-2 hr	3/4"over	45-60 min
Kidney Beans	3	1.5-2 hr	1/2"over	45-60 min
Navy Beans	2	1.5-2 hr	1/2"over	45-60 min
Pinto Beans	3	2-2.5 hr	1/2"over	45-60 min
Chickpeas (Garbanzos)	4	1.5-3 hr	1/2"over	75-90 min
Azuki Beans	3	2-2.5 hr	1/2"over	45-60 min
Soy Beans	3-4	3-4 hr	3/4"over	50-75 min

Savory Garbanzo Beans

- 1 C garbanzo beans
- 1 Tbsp miso
- 3 C water
- optional 3" strip of konbu

Wash garbanzo beans and soak in water 6 to 12 hours. If you don't soak them, use a little more water and cook a little longer. If using konbu, rinse it and place it in the bottom of the pot. Place beans in a pressure cooker or pot. Add water to cover beans 1/2" over the level of the beans for a pressure cooker, slightly more for a regular pot. Dilute miso in the water. Pressure cook for 35 to 40 minutes or boil in a pot for 1-1/2 to 2 hours (in either case, bring to boil on high then turn to low heat).

Black Beans Mexicana

(Contributed by Kathy Cain)

- 2 C black beans
- 5 C water
- 1 medium onion, diced
- 1 tsp sea salt
- 1 tsp cumin seeds
- 1 or 2 bay leaf

Wash beans and soak for 4 to 6 hours before cooking if you have time. If you don't soak them, use a little more water and cook a little longer. Place onions in the bottom of a pot and add beans and water. Bring to a boil and add bay leaf, cover and reduce heat to low and simmer for 1-1/2 hours. Add sea salt 30 to 45 minutes before serving and add cumin just before cooking is done.

Lentil Salad Sandwich

• leftover, cooked lentils
• 1 small onion, minced
• 1 small carrot, matchstick
• 1 small stalk celery, diced
• tamari to taste
• lettuce leaves
• sesame oil (optional)
• whole grain bread or sprouted grain bread

Saute onions in very small amount of sesame oil (or water) until transparent. Add celery and carrot. Slightly mash some of the lentils and add to the vegetables. Season to taste with tamari. Allow mixture to cool. Toast or bread, place a lettuce leaf, then mashed lentil mixture, then another lettuce leaf, then top slice of bread. Apply slight pressure and slice and serve. Crunchy, organic pickles go good with these sandwiches.

Tempeh cutlets

Tempeh is a soy bean product that is an excellent meat substitute. It is lightly fermented so that the "beany" flavor is eliminated. It is available in most health food stores

• 1 piece 1/4 to 1/2" thick piece of tempeh
• 1 Tbsp low-sodium tamari
• 1 tsp ginger juice
• 2 Tbsp water

Place tempeh in a bakeware dish that has a cover, marinate in the tamari with ginger juice and water, and bake at 350 degrees for about 25 min. This can be served as a simple bean dish with rice or potatoes or can be delicious if used in a sandwich.

Sloppy Jim (n)

- 2 C cooked beans (canned or pre-cooked beans such as pinto beans)
- 2/3 C tomatoes or prepared no-oil pasta sauce
- 1 onion, finely chopped
- 1/2 tsp garlic powder or 1 clove garlic, crushed
- 1 tsp soy sauce
- 1 tsp blackstrap molasses or barley malt
- Sea salt

Saute the onion in water and the soy sauce until slightly translucent. Place all ingredients in blender and puree. Heat and spread on bread and top with lettuce, sprouts, and other greens and sprinkle chopped olives or other condiments.

Jerry's Burritos (n)

(Contributed by Jerry Smith)

- 2 pkg whole wheat tortillas or chapatis
- 2 onions, chopped
- 3 cloves garlic, crushed
- 28 oz can tomatoes
- 2 cans black beans (15 oz can), drained
- 1 C frozen corn
- 8 oz package 5-grain tempeh crumbled or diced
- 1 Tbsp chili powder
- 1 Tbsp chili con carne seasoning
- 2 tsp cumin
- 2 tsp coriander
- 1/4 tsp cayenne

Saute onions and garlic in 1/2 C water until soft. Add tomatoes, beans corn, tempeh and seasonings. Cook, uncovered for 30 minutes, stirring occasionally. Spread a line of this mixture down the center of a whole wheat tortilla and roll it up. You may add shredded lettuce, chopped raw vegetables or salsa if you like.

Bean Tacos (n)

- 1 pkg taco shells
- 1 bowl shredded lettuce
- 2 C chopped tomatoes
- 1 C chopped olives
- 1 bowl low-fat or no-fat refried beans (can be bought in most stores)

Slightly heat taco shells, fill with heated beans, then add other ingredients. Serve with salsa (can be bought in most natural foods stores) . Or make your own salsa using: chopped fresh tomatoes, garlic, onion, cilantro, chile pepper, sliced tomatoes, salt, and liquid from tomatoes; and mixing together in a bowl.

Quick Chili (n)

(Contributed by Ann Tang)

There are several excellent canned vegetarian chilies on the market. If you don't feel like cooking tonight, you can use one of these, cook the brown rice, and you have dinner. However, if you don't have access to a good vegetarian chili, here's one for you:
(cooked beans needed)

- 1/2 C water
- 2 onions chopped
- 1 green pepper, chopped
- 1 stalk celery, chopped
- 1 clove garlic, crushed
- 2 (16 oz) cans tomato, cut up
- 4 C cooked kidney beans (canned or from fresh)
- 2 Tbsp chili powder
- 2 tsp ground cumin

Place water, onions, green pepper, celery, and garlic in a medium sauce pan and saute over high heat for 3-4 minutes. Add remaining ingredients, bring to a boil, reduce heat and cook gently for another 25 minutes or so to blend flavors. Stir occasionally.

Serve this over brown rice or baked potatoes. You can use other kinds of beans such as black beans, or white beans.

Baked Beans (n)

- 4 C cooked beans (e.g. white beans, or pinto beans)
- 1/4 C water
- 2/3 C tomato sauce
- 1 tsp chili powder
- 1-1/2 Tbsp molasses
- 1/2 tsp dry mustard

Water saute the onions in a large pan or wok. Then add the beans and other spices, and stir. Reduce the heat to low and cook for about 30 minutes.

Azuki Beans

- 3" piece konbu
- 1 C azuki beans
- 2-3 C water
- bay leaf
- 1/4-1/2 tsp sea salt

Rinse konbu off under running water. Place konbu in sauce pan, then azuki beans, which have been sorted for stones and rinsed and drained. Add water, cover and bring to a boil. Reduce flame, add bay leaf, and simmer about 1-1/2 hours or until tender. Add sea salt and simmer for 5 more minutes. Serve.

Azuki Beans with Squash

- 2 C Azuki beans
- 1 Medium butternut or acorn squash; or Hokkaido or Kabocha Pumpkin
- 1/2 tsp sea salt or 1 Tbsp miso
- Optional, 1 strip konbu 6" long

Sort azuki beans for small stones and wash. Soak the beans 4 to 6 hours if you have time. If not, use a little more water and cook a little longer. If using konbu, rinse it, soak it in water till soft and place it in the bottom of the pot. Scrub and cut the squash into 1" cubes and add to pot. Add washed beans to pot and add water (about 4-5 cups) to cover squash. Bring to boil and turn down to low and cook for 1-1/2 to 2 hours. Add salt or miso about 15 minutes before done.

STEWS

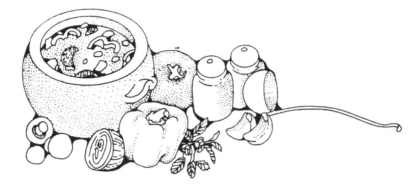

Stews are especially good during cool weather. In addition, they can be high in EMI and very satisfying while you lose weight. You can use a variety of solid vegetables such as carrots, turnips, potatoes, onions, and the like. However, as in casseroles, they do take some time to prepare.

Ann's Vegetarian Stew (n)

(Contributed by Ann Tang)

- 4 cloves garlic, minced
- 1 round onion, chopped
- 2 C water
- 2 stalks celery, chopped
- 2 carrots, cubed
- 1 bell pepper, cubed
- 1 large can whole tomatoes, chopped
- 2 fresh tomatoes, chopped (optional)
- 1 turnip, cubed
- 1 sweet potato, yam or 1/2 New Zealand pumpkin, cubed
- 2 potatoes, cubed

- 2 C cauliflower, cut in pieces
- 2 C broccoli, cut in pieces
- 1 zucchini, cubed
- 1 C uncooked dry beans (black turtle, kidney, navy, pinto, lentils, etc.)
  or 1 can each kidney and garbanzo beans
- 1 box frozen lima beans
- 1 box frozen corn or 1 can unsalted corn
- 1/2 C organic barley
- 1 Tbsp cilantro, chopped
- 1/4 C apple juice (or, to taste)
- 1/2 lemon (juice only) (or, to taste)
- 1/4 tsp red pepper flakes, optional

Saute garlic and onions in 1 cup water until transparent. Add carrots, celery and bell pepper and cook for 3-5 minutes. Add canned tomatoes, with juice, and the optional fresh tomatoes. Bring to a boil. Add beans, if using dry type, turnip and all potatoes, as well as New Zealand pumpkin, and simmer 30 minutes or until beans are tender. Add barley, beans, (if using canned) corn, cauliflower, broccoli, zucchini, lima beans, and apple/lemonjuice. Simmer 30 minutes and stir occasionally.

Mixed Vegetable Curry (n)

- 1 round onion
- 3 cloves garlic
- 1 stalks celery
- 2 carrots
- 2 potatoes
- 1 chopped green pepper
- 1 C chopped broccoli
- 1 C chopped cauliflower
- 1/2 C sliced fresh mushrooms
- 1 Tbsp curry powder
- 1 tsp tumeric
- 1/2 tsp coriander
- 1 tsp ground cumin
- 1/4 tsp dry mustard
- 1/4 tsp chili powder
- 2 T whole wheat flour

Chop onions, and peppers into small pieces. Slice carrots, cut celery, broccoli, and cauliflower into medium size pieces, and cut potatoes into chunks. Place onions with crushed garlic in a saucepan and saute with water and a little soy sauce until translucent. Add spices, and 1 T flour and saute for a few minutes adding more water and stirring to form a sauce. Add carrots, celery and potatoes, cover and cook for 25 minutes. Add rest of ingredients and cook another 15 minutes. Add soy sauce or salt to taste. Serve over brown rice or as a filling for baked potatoes or with whole wheat chapati (Indian flat bread).

Nishime (Japanese) Stew

- 2 to 3 strips konbu
- 5 to 6 six- to eight-inch long shiitake mushrooms
- 4 or more of the following: 1 onion, 2 carrots, 1 daikon (turnip), 1 burdock root, 1 small taro.
- 1 lotus root.

Soak konbu in warm water (save the water), then slice into 3" x 1/2" strips. Tie each konbu strip into a knot. Wash and dice onions into 1/2 - 3/4" cubes. Begin soaking shiitake mushrooms in warm water. Cut daikon, carrots, burdock, lotus root, and/or taro into large 1/2 to 1-inch pieces. Brush a pot with sesame oil and place cubed onions at the bottom of the pot. Take shiitake mushrooms (save the soaking water) and slice into quarters or 1-inch to 2-inch pieces. Place shiitake on the onions, then the konbu knots, and then the rest of the vegetables. Add the soaking water of the konbu and shiitake and add enough water to the pot to almost cover vegetables. Bring to boil and simmer for 30 to 35 minutes or until daikon is tender (translucent) and add Tamari or soy sauce to taste and simmer for 5 more minutes.

Beans and Carrot Stew (n)

(Contributed by Anne Tang)

- 1 C pink beans
- 1 C black turtle beans
- 5 fresh tomatoes, chopped
- 1 bell pepper, chopped
- 1 Anaheim pepper, chopped
- 3 stalks celery, chopped
- 6 large carrots, diced
- 1/2 round onion, chopped
- 6 sprigs parsley, chopped
- 1-1/2 Tbsp chili powder
- 1/2 tsp paprika
- 1/2 tsp oregano
- 1/2 tsp summer savory
- 1/2 bay leaf
- 1 clove garlic, minced

Saute garlic and onion in 2 cups water until transparent. Add tomatoes and beans and simmer 1 hour. Add remainder of ingredients and simmer another 30-45 minutes.

Excellent with brown rice or over a baked potato. Freezes well.

Chickpea (garbanzo) A La King

(Adapted from Country Life Vegetarian Cookbook, used by permission)

Saute in 4 Tbsp water:
- 1 medium chopped onion
- 1 4-oz can mushrooms (about 1 C of each)

Blend until smooth:
- 3 C water
- 1/4 C cashew pieces
- 4 Tbsp sesame seeds

• 3 Tbsp McKay's Chicken Seasoning, or substitutes
(most stores now carry something similar)
• 1/2 C whole wheat flour

When smooth, add to onions and mushrooms, then add:
• 1-1/2 C frozen green peas
• 2 oz pimentos (chopped)
• 1 C (15 oz) garbanzo beans

Cook until thickened, stirring carefully to keep from scorching.
Serve over brown rice or sprouted wheat toast or whole wheat
flat noodles or fold cooked noodles into sauce and bake about
20 minutes at 350°.

Sukiyaki

• watercress
• won bok cabbage
• carrots, sliced into matchskicks
• mung bean sprouts
• bamboo shoots
• shiitake mushrooms
• round onions and or green onions
• cellophane noodles (available in oriental section of markets)
• maple syrup
• low sodium soy sauce
• 1 C Water
• 2 C boiling water (to soak noodles)
• tofu

Rinse 6 to 8 half-dollar sized shiitake mushrooms and soak in
water. Save the water for sukiyaki stock. Saute slivered
onions and slivered mushrooms in water and a dash to a tsp of
sesame oil. Sprinkle some sea salt to prevent sticking. Add
mushroom water and season to taste with low-sodium soy sauce
and maple syrup. Add bamboo shoots to mixture, bring to boil
and simmer at a low boil. Add soaked and drained cellophane
noodles to mixture. Sprinkle julienned carrots. Layer watercress bean sprouts and won bok and cover and allow upper lay-
ers of vegetables to be steamed.

Ann's Garbanzo Casserole (n)

(Contributed by Ann Tang)

- 1/2 lb cooked garbanzo beans
- 1 8oz can whole tomatoes
- 1 Onion cut into 1/2" chunks
- 1 carrot, sliced
- 1 tsp Basil

Soak garbanzo beans overnight in water to cover, or bring to boil, remove from heat and let rest for one hour. Saute onions and carrots in 1 C water. Add soaked beans and tomatoes. Add more water to cover and add the basil. Bring to a boil, cover and simmer for at least 2 hours until garbanzos are tender.

SIDE DISHES

SALADS

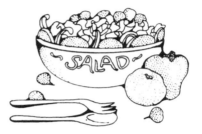

Salads are one of the simplest ways to eat leafy greens and other great high EMI foods. One of the problems, however, is that most salad dressings are very high in fat and oil which, of course, is the lowest in EMI of all foods and can easily ruin the weight-loss value of a salad. The trick is to use salad dressings that are medium to high in EMI and contain little or no oil. You can purchase ready-made no-oil dressing at the health food store. There are even prepared dry dressing mixes you can make just by adding water. If you want to make some dressings from scratch, look at the section on sauces and dressings.

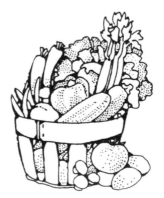

LEAFY GREENS

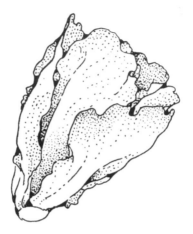

Leafy greens are a fundamental part of the Eat More Diet.   I recommend eating large servings of these foods. These are not only the highest in EMI and will help induce weight loss, but the dark green varieties are among the best sources of certain minerals.   Notably, they are generally high in calcium and some of them are also high in iron.

Steamed Greens

- 2 large bunches greens of your choice. (Collards, kale, mustard greens, daikon greens, or a combination of two)
- water

Wash the greens thoroughly, and chop into bite-sized pieces. Pour about 1-1/2 cups water into a pan, add the greens, cover, and bring to a boil. Reduce flame and cook over low flame until just tender but still bright green. Remove to serving dish right away to retain bright green color.   Serve with tofu dressing described in "Dressings" section.

Steamed Collard Greens With Carrots

(See Day 5 recipes)

Steamed Cabbage

(See Day 2 recipes)

Steamed Collard Greens

(See Day 5 recipes)

Steamed Daikon Greens

- 1 bunch daikon greens
- 1/2 - 1 C water

Wash the greens and slice on the diagonal into bite-sized pieces. Place water into saucepan, add the greens, cover, and bring to a boil. Reduce the flame immediately and simmer until just tender but still bright green. Remove the lid and serve greens into serving dish to retain the bright green color.

Parboiled Greens

- 1 Large bunch each, kale/collards/turnip greens
- 2 C water

Wash greens thoroughly and slice on the diagonal into bite-sized pieces. Place in 2 cups water and cover and bring to a boil. Reduce flame and simmer for 10 to 15 minutes or until greens are just tender but still bright green. Drain and remove to a serving dish to retain bright green color.

Steamed Greens With Carrots

- 2 big bunches collard greens
- 1 large carrot, sliced on the diagonal
- 1/2-1 C water
- pinch sea salt

Wash the greens, drain, stack leaves, slice down the center, lengthwise. Then stack halves on top of each other and cut on the diagonal into bite-sized pieces. Pour water into a pan, add pinch sea salt, add the greens, then the carrots on top of the greens, cover and bring to a boil. Reduce the flame and simmer just until tender and greens are bright green (approximately 5 to 7 minutes). Don't stir. Remove to a serving bowl.

SQUASH AND OTHER SOLID VEGETABLES

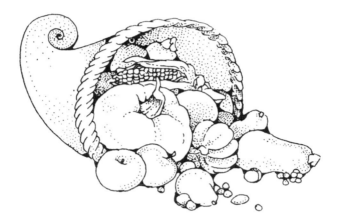

One of the best kept secrets in weight-loss cuisine is the squash. It is high in EMI and provides a surprisingly tasty and versatile food. It is easy to prepare and most varieties are high in beta-carotene, which is likely to provide some protection against cancer.

Summer Squash and Onions

This is a simple dish that is surprisingly tasty.

- 1 medium summer squash
- 1 medium onion

Scrub squash (cut into 1/2-inch rounds). Slice onions into crescents then saute in small amount of water until translucent, add squash, stir occasionally. Cover and cook over low flame until tender.

Squash Deluxe

- 1 Buttercup or acorn squash, or kabocha pumpkin
- 1 Tbsp miso
- 1 tsp maple syrup (or other sweetener)
- Water

Scrub squash until clean and cut into quarters. Place in 1" of water and cook in pressure cooked by bringing it to pressure at high heat and cooking at low heat for about 2 to 3 minutes. (If not using a pressure cooker, boil in a covered pot for about 15 minutes). Test with barbecue stick to see if it is tender. Cook a little longer if it is not. Then cut into 1 to 2 inch chunks. Mix in a separate bowl the miso, and maple syrup in 1/4 C water. Add to the water in the pot with the squash and bring to boil and simmer with pot uncovered for 5 to 10 minutes. Serve on a platter garnished with parsley sprigs.

Baked Butternut Squash

- 1 medium large butternut squash
- Pinch sea salt
- 1/2 C water

Scrub squash, cut in half, remove seeds, and cut again into quarters. Add water to baking dish, add sea salt, place pieces of squash in dish, cover and bake in 350 degree oven for 45 minutes or until squash tests tender with toothpick. Serve on a platter.

Steamed Greens and Summer Squash

- 2 big bunches kale greens, washed and chopped
- 2-3 med. summer squash
- Pinch of sea salt
- Water

Pour about 1-1/2 inches of water into a pan, add a pinch of sea salt, then the greens, then the squash. Cover the pan and bring to a boil. Reduce flame to a medium heat and cook for 5 to 8 minutes or until greens are just bright green and tender. Remove from pan and serve.

Steamed Chard with Potatoes (n)

• 2 clove garlic crushed
• 1 bunch whiter or red swiss chard cut into pieces
• 2 C water
• 2 white or red potatoes chunked
• Low sodium soy sauce

Place water, chard, and garlic into saucepan, bring to boil, turn down to simmer, cover, and cook for 10 minutes. Add potatoes, then stir and cover. Cook for 25 to 30 minutes. Add soy sauce to taste. For variation, add 1 to 2 C cooked pinto beans or black turtle beans.

Grated Zucchini with Onion

• 1 med. onion, minced
• 3 C grated zucchini
• 1/2 tsp sesame oil (optional)
• 1/4-1/2 tsp sea salt
• 1/2 tsp lemon or orange peel, grated fine or 1 tsp lemon juice.

Saute minced onion with cover until transparent. Add grated zucchini and salt and saute without cover for 10 minutes. Serve with finely grated citrus peel or juice.

Summer Squash and Mushroom with Konbu

• 1 medium summer squash
• 5 shiitake mushrooms (black mushrooms)
• 8" piece konbu
• 1 Tbsp maple syrup
• 1/2 onion
• 1 garlic clove
• water
• low sodium soy sauce

Rinse mushrooms lightly and soak in water to cover mushrooms. Save the soaking water as soup stock. Soak an 8" piece of konbu in water. Slice shiitake mushrooms into 1/4" wide strips after soaked. Slice konbu into roughly 1" x 1/2" pieces. Slice a half onion vertically into crescents. Peel squash with potato peeler, slice and scoop out seeds. Then slice into 1" pieces. In heated saucepan, place 1 tsp sesame oil. Sprinkle a little sea salt to prevent sticking because oil is so little. Add mushrooms, onions and 1 clove crushed garlic and saute. Add mushroom liquid to cover mushrooms and allow to boil. Add 1 Tbsp maple syrup. Add low sodium soy sauce to taste. Add squash and konbu and simmer with cover until squash is tender (about 15 minutes).

Steamed Vegetables

Broccoli, cauliflower, carrots and snow peas, steamed and served, make a wonderful compliment to any of the dishes above.

Spaghetti Squash

If you have never tried spaghetti squash, do yourself a favor and buy one the next time you go to the grocery store. It is a fun food and one that has a pleasantly mild flavor. It actually looks like pale orange spaghetti noodles.

Scrub squash well and place in oven which has been preheated to 350°. Bake until squash tests tender with a skewer. Remove to a cutting board, cut in half, length-wise, remove seeds from the center. Cut each half into two pieces, length-wise. Take a fork and shred inside meat of the squash length-wise until all the squash is free of the skin. It will resemble strands of cooked spaghetti. You can even pour pasta sauce of your choice over it and eat it like spaghetti.

Rice "Gravy" Over
Steamed Vegetables
on Toast

Steam any seasonal veggies of choice. Puree leftover cooked brown rice in a blender with enough water to make a thick gravy. Use whatever amount is necessary to feed number of people being served. Heat "gravy," flavor with miso, and serve over veggies on toast.

Steamed Broccoli and Cauliflower with Sesame Salt

- several bunches broccoli
- small to medium head cauliflower

Wash and cut broccoli and cauliflower into flowerettes. Steam in 1/2inch of water in covered pan until just tender. Remove from steam to cool.

Broccoli with Mushrooms

- several large bunches of broccoli
- 1 lb. fresh mushrooms
- water

Wash and cut broccoli into flowerettes. Peel the outer layer of stem part off and cut stem on the diagonal, 1/4-inch slices. Place in pan with 2 inches of water in the bottom. Wash and slice mushrooms in thin slices and place on top of the broccoli. Cover and bring to a boil. Reduce flame and simmer for 5 to 8 minutes or just until broccoli is bright green and tender. Serve.

ROOT VEGETABLES

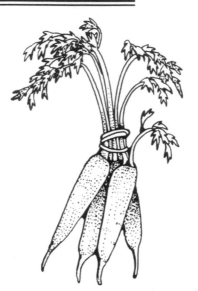

I put root vegetables in a different category because they are cooked slightly differently. Root vegetables include familiar ones such as potatoes (which are nightshades) carrots, onions and turnips, and unfamiliar ones such as burdock and lotus root. They are medium to high in EMI and quite satisfying. Here are some examples of root vegetables that are hearty and an excellent complement to your other dishes.

Steamed Sweet Potato or Yams

I rediscovered how delicious sweet potatoes are when I conducted the original trial of the Wai`anae Diet Program at the Wai`anae Coast Comprehensive Health Center in 1989 (in which the weight-loss effects of the traditional Hawaiian diet were demonstrated). Sweet potatoes and yams were staple foods of the traditional Hawaiians, and they are simple and simply delicious by themselves. They don't have to be eaten only at Thanksgiving. They are great at any meal or even as snacks.

* Sweet Potatoes or Yams
* Water

Place whole sweet potatoes in steamer with 1" water and steam for approximately 15 minutes or until fork tender. Slice and serve.

Taro

Taro is a root vegetable that most people are not acquainted with but this was the primary staple of ancient Hawai'i and most of the rest of Polynesia, and is found on all continents including Asia, Africa, and the Americas. It must be cooked well or the oxalate crystals will make your mouth itch. It can be eaten alone or with stews.

Preparation: Place in steamer and steam for two to three hours (depending on the size of the taro) until fork tender. Then scrape the skin off, slice and serve. Pressure cooking for 1-1/2 to 2 hours is another way to prepare taro.

Baked Potatoes (n)

Bake one potato per serving, top with mushroom gravy (see spaghetti recipe above or mushroom marinara sauce).

Hashbrowns (n)

Steam six large potatoes, when done let cool, then shred. Form into pancakes and cook in lightly olive-oiled skillet till golden brown.

Potato Presto (n)

* 1 onions, sliced vertically into crescents
* 1 carrot, thinly sliced diagonally
* 4 white potatoes, thinly sliced
* 1 C of mushrooms, sliced
* 1 large handful greens of your choice such as kale or won bok
* 1 Tbsp low-sodium soy sauce
* 1/2 C water

In a pan with a cover, saute the onions and carrots in 1/4 C
water and a little soy sauce until onions are translucent. Add
the potatoes and more water if necessary, then cover the pan so
the vegetables can steam. Steam for about 15 minutes, remov-
ing the cover to stir occasionally. Add the mushrooms, greens
and the soy sauce and cook uncovered about ten minutes
longer, stirring often.

Carrots and Green Beans

• 1 lb. green beans
• 2 large carrots
• water
• pinch sea salt

Wash green beans and slice in 1-inch diagonal pieces if they
are long beans and slice carrots into 1/4" diagonal slices.
Place 2 inches of water in pan, add beans and carrots, and
pinch of sea salt. Cover and bring to a boil. Reduce flame and
simmer for 5 to 10 minutes or just until veggies are tender but
beans are still bright green. Serve with or without a sauce.

Burdock Root

Burdock root is a long thin root vegetable that is used in the
Orient. It has a color similar to potatoes but is crunchier and
has a hearty but mellow flavor.

• 3 fresh burdock, cut into matchsticks
• 1 medium carrot, cut into matchsticks
• 1/4 tsp sesame oil
• 2 Tbsp low-sodium soy sauce

Saute burdock in water and oil in a covered pan for about 10
minutes. Stir occasionally. Add carrot and saute well. Add
1/2 cup of water around the edge of the pan, simmer until about
half done, then season with soy sauce. Remove cover when
vegetables are tender. Add soy sauce to taste.

Turnips (daikon) with Greens and Konbu

- turnips, with tops
- water
- sliced konbu
- low sodium soy sauce or tamari

Wash turnips (daikon) and tops (or other leafy greens if daikon tops are unavailable). Slice the turnips into chunks and place in a pot with a strip of soaked, sliced konbu which has been simmered in water to cover till tender. Add 1/2 to 1cup of water, cover pot, and cook for 10 to 15 minutes or until daikon is tender throughout. (Add more water if necessary.) Add the chopped greens and after 1 to 2 minutes sprinkle with shoyu, then steam an additional 2 to 3 minutes.

SEA VEGETABLE DISHES
SEA VEGETABLES

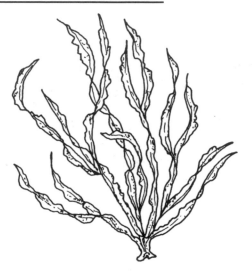

This is a wonderful category of high-calcium, non-dairy food that we should all learn to prepare and eat regularly. This is one of the secrets to the health of the longest-lived people in the world, the Japanese. Actually, this food was eaten around the world in the past, including Ireland where they ate dulse. Seafood without cholesterol is what I call sea vegetables, (or seaweed as it is commonly known). Ounce for ounce, seaweed has more calcium than milk and more iron than beef. What's even better is that it is very low in fat and has no cholesterol. The only drawbacks are that it is quite salty if you don't rinse it, and also, most people are unfamiliar with seaweed as a food. But it is considered to be a delicacy in much of Asia. So try some of these recipes and make them part of your regular meals. You may wonder why nobody ever before told you about such a delicious and nutritious food.

DULSE

Dulse is a seaweed that was eaten in its raw, dried form in the British Isles. It is available as "dulse chips" in health food stores in Boston, Connecticut and Maine, and recently I see they've been imported to Honolulu. These chips may be available elsewhere as well.

NORI

Nori as the wrapper of sushi or "California Rolls" is often the the average American's first taste of sea vegetables. It is available in health food stores and is great for wrapping rice dishes, including leftover fried rice. Some varieties can be eaten plain as a snack like chips or crackers, in the same way dulse is eaten.

WAKAME

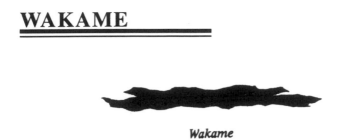

Wakame

Wakame is a leafy sea vegetable often used in soup. One of the easiest ways to eat it is to buy "wakame flakes" and toss them in a soup that you are making. Miso soup is a logical choice but it will work in just about any soup. It quickly absorbs water and the soup's flavor, blends right in. You will be amazed that when wet, it swells to about five times its dry size. One neat trick I use is to carry it to the restaurant and toss a small handful in my soup.

Wakame is also delicious as a side-dish in its own right. You can simply soak wakame in water and drain to remove the sodium, and you have a simple fresh green to use as a side dish or as a high-calcium addition to any salad. You can also cook it with other vegetables, to make delicious side-dishes. Here are a few examples:

Wakame Vinaigrette

- 1 oz Wakame
- (Optional) 1/2 - 1 C Sliced cucumbers, julienned carrots, sliced radish or daikon or any combination)
- Sushi vinegar to taste (available in oriental food section) or use brown rice vinegar mixed with a sweetener such as barley malt and a little sea salt to taste.

Rinse and soak the wakame in water. Thinly slice or julienne the cucumbers, carrots and/or any other vegetables. Mix with the sauce, let stand for 10 minutes so the flavor mixes with the vegetables. Serve as a cool, tangy side vegetable.

Wakame with Onions

- 1 oz wakame (dry weight)
- 1 - 2 medium-sized onion
- water
- low-sodium soy sauce, about one Tbsp

Rinse, and soak the wakame in water until tender, then slice into roughly one-inch pieces. Peel and slice onions vertically into crescents. Place onions in a pot, then cover with wakame. Add water to nearly cover the wakame. Bring the mixture to a boil, and reduce the heat to low. Simmer for about 15 minutes to taste. Season with low-sodium soy sauce to taste, and cook for 10 minutes longer.

Wakame with Carrots (or other vegetables)

- 1 oz wakame (dried)
- 1-1/2 to 2 C large chunks of carrots (or other vegetables such as cauliflower, turnips, daikon, celery burdock or lotus root).
- water to cover vegetables
- 2 - 3 tsp low-sodium soy sauce
- (optional) cilantro, scallions, chives or parsley for garnish

Rinse, and soak wakame. Slice into large pieces. Put the carrots (or other vegetables) in a pot, and add water to half cover the carrots. Bring to a boil, cover and reduce the heat to low.

Simmer until the carrots are nearly done (about 20 - 30 minutes. Adjust cooking time for other vegetables). Then add the wakame and low-sodium soy sauce to taste and simmer until carrots are done. Garnish.

KONBU (Kelp or Laminaria)

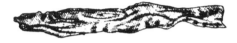

Kombu

Konbu is a hearty sea vegetable that can be used as a food by itself or as a base for soup stock. It is thick and hard to cut until it is soaked. In traditional Japanese and Chinese dishes, it is soaked, rinsed, cut into 2 inch by 4 to 6 inch strips and tied into a knot for bite-sized side dishes or to cook in a stew (see the recipe for "nishime" in the stew section above). It also goes well with other vegetables (see squash mushroom konbu above). As with other sea vegetables, it is rich in iron and calcium.

Konbu with Carrots & Onion

- 1 piece konbu, (about 10") or 2 medium pieces (about 6")
- water
- 1 medium carrot
- 1 round onion
- low-sodium soy sauce to taste (about 1-2 Tbsp)

Rinse and soak the konbu for 4 minutes and save the water. Slice konbu strip length-wise, then cut into 1-inch-long pieces. Slice carrots diagonally into 1-inch chunks and the onions vertically into large pieces. Place the sliced konbu in a pot and on top of the konbu add the onions and carrots. Then add enough soaking water to half cover the vegetables, and bring to a boil. Simmer for 20 - 25 minutes at medium low heat. Season with low-sodium soy sauce to taste and simmer about 10 more minutes.

Konbu Mushroom Dried Daikon

- 2 medium pieces konbu 6 - 8"
- one handful dried daikon
- 3 - 5 shiitake mushrooms (depending on size) or other mushrooms
- water
- low-sodium soy sauce to taste

Rinse, and soak the konbu and save the water. Slice konbu into 1" pieces. Soak, stem, and slice mushrooms. Place the konbu in a pot with the shiitake. Soak and slice the dried daikon and place on top. Add the soaking water of the konbu to just cover daikon and bring to a boil. Cover and simmer about 30 minutes at low to medium low. Season with a little low-sodium soy sauce to taste and simmer until remaining liquid is nearly gone.

HIJIKI

Hijiki is a delicious string-like or thread-like sea vegetable that is very high in calcium and iron (as are virtually all sea vegetables). It is virtually interchangable with arame (described next) although it takes longer to cook hijiki. It has a strong ocean aroma that disappears after it is cooked off so don't let the initial fragrance prevent you from using it. It is delicious with other vegetables. Remember that the Hijiki and arame recipes are interchangable.

Hijiki with Onions (or other vegetables)

* 1 oz hijiki (or arame) dry weight
* 1/4 - 1/2 tsp sesame oil
* 1 -2 onions (or other vegetables such as carrots, burdock root, lotus root, or tofu.)
* water
* low-sodium soy sauce to taste (about 2-3 Tbsp)
* (optional) a dash of sweetener such as barley malt

Wash and rinse the hijiki in a strainer or colander. After washing, be sure to place in a separate bowl to drain to eliminate any sand that may be present. Then soak hijiki for about 10 minutes. While soaking, slice onion vertically into thin crescents. Lighly oil a frying pan, and heat it. Add the onions and a little water and saute for 2 to 3 minutes. Place the hijiki on top of the onions and add water to cover the onions. Bring to a boil, turn the heat to low, then add a small amount of low-sodium soy sauce. Cover and simmer for about 40 minutes (depending on the vegetable). Add soy sauce to taste. Simmer for another 15 minutes, or until the liquid is almost gone.

ARAME

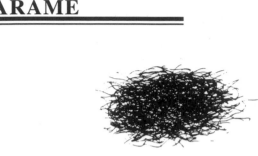

Arame

Arame (pronounced "are-ah-meh") appears to be another "stringy" sea vegetable like hijiki when you buy it, but it is actually a flat seaweed that is finely sliced to its stringy appearance. Because it is sliced, the cut edges are exposed and it therefore cooks slightly faster than hijiki. It is nonetheless interchangable in hijiki recipes. However, It can be used in soups and pilafs more easily than hijiki.

Arame with Corn (or carrots)

- 1 oz arame (dry weight)
- 1/2 tsp sesame oil
- 1 C onions sliced vertically into thin crescents
- water
- 2 - 3 Tbsp low-sodium soy sauce
- 1 - 2C fresh corn kernels (or 1 C julienned carrots)

Wash and drain the arame. After washing, be sure to place in a separate bowl to eliminate any sand that may be present. Lighly oil a frying pan, add a little water and heat it. Saute the onions for 1 to 2 minutes, stirring gently. (If using carrots, add julienned carrots at this time on the onions). Place the arame on top and enough water to cover the onions. Add a little low-sodium soy sauce. Cover and bring to a boil, then turn flame to low and simmer for about 20 minutes. Place the corn on top and a little more soy sauce to taste. Simmer for another 10 or so minutes or until the water is nearly gone.

SAUCES, GRAVIES, DRESSINGS
DIPS

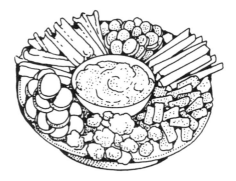

Fancy Hummus (Garbanzo Beans Spread)

- 1 C Garbanzo beans (if using canned beans, cut down on miso and umeboshi as the beans are already a little salty)
- 3-4 inches of konbu
- 2 C water
- 1 clove garlic chopped
- 1 tsp miso (optional)
- 2 Tbsp tahini
- 1 Tbsp minced onion
- 2-3 umeboshi plum

Wash beans and pick out stones. Soak 8 to 12 hours. Pour off soaking water and add 2 cups of fresh water. Break or cut konbu into 1-inch pieces. Boil for 2-1/2 hours or pressure cook for 50 minutes (bring to pressure on high heat then simmer at low) then pour off and save the water. Place beans in blender with rest of ingredients and blend with saved water poured in a little at a time until creamy.

This is delicious with rice cakes, natural low-salt corn chips and homemade "chips" made by toasting corn tortillas, chapati or pita bread cut into triangles. Simply cut the pita bread or chapati into chip-sized pieces and place in your toaster oven. Watch them because they may burn if toasted too long. When they are a nice toasty color and aroma, place them on a plate and serve with this delicious bean dip or salsa for dipping.

Simple Hummus

- 1 C cooked garbanzo beans
- 2-3 Tbsp lemon juice
- 1 Tbsp minced onion
- 1 clove crushed garlic
- 1 tsp cumin
- low Sodium soy sauce (or salt) and pepper to taste
- enough water to keep a thick moist dip consistency

If using dry garbanzo beans, cook as described above or use the bean cooking chart in this book. You may use pre-cooked canned beans instead if you wish. Mash beans and mix ingredients together.

Tofu Dip

(See "Tofu Dressing")

DRESSINGS

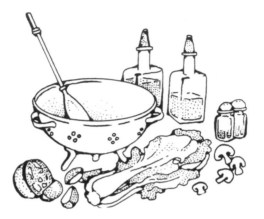

For salad dressings, the easiest way is to purchase a bottled "no-oil dressing. It is very easy to get fooled by dressings that boldly state "no cholesterol" or "low fat". However, since no vegetable oil ever had cholesterol in it, a vegetable oil based dressing can have as much as 100% fat, and usually has around 90% fat.

Packaged No-Oil Dressings

You can easily make your own fresh no-oil dressings by purchasing a packet of salad dressing mix. Just make sure it says "no-oil" on it. Simply follow the instructions and add water, vinegar and whatever else is suggested for the mix and use fresh on your salad.

Tofu Dressing

This is one of the most versatile dressings to use with steamed vegetables because you can add just about any of your favorite spices and ingredients to it.

- 1/2 block of tofu, firm is preferable
- 1 clove garlic, minced

- 1 Tbsp tahini
- 1 tsp miso
- 1 Tbsp lemon juice
- (optional) other ingredients of your choice such as parsley, mustard, curry powder, umeboshi plum.

Blend all ingredients until creamy smooth. Be careful. Tofu spoils easily so if you want it to keep for an extra day, steam it for 3 minutes before blending and refrigerate dressing immediately.

Tofu Mayonnaise

(Contributed by Elaine French)

- 1/2 block tofu or 1 (10oz) block Mori-Nu tofu (firm)
- 1 clove garlic
- 1 Tbsp parsley flakes
- 1 Tbsp lemon juice
- 3/4 tsp ground coriander
- 2 Tbsp low-sodium soy sauce

Place all ingredients in a blender or food processor and blend until smooth. Add a little water if necessary. Be careful. Tofu spoils easily so if you want it to keep for an extra day, steam it for 3 minutes before blending and refrigerate dressing immediately.

Dijon Dressing

- 2 tsp Dijon mustard
- 2 Tbsp lemon juice
- 2 Tbsp vinegar
- 1 clove garlic crushed or 1 tsp garlic powder
- 1/4 tsp sea salt or 1 tsp low sodium soy sauce to taste
- pepper to taste (fresh ground if possible)
- (optional) 1/2 tsp honey or barley malt, 1/2 tsp onion powder, 1/2 tsp dill

Mix ingredients well and use on salads, steamed vegetables, pastas, potato dishes, or dipping sauce.

GRAVIES AND SAUCES

Gravies help to enhance the flavor of your meals. While most of us are used to having gravies made from animal fats, here are examples of gravies that are better alternatives. They can make a very simple dish of vegetables, beans, noodles or grains very special.

Gravies can be very simple and require a few common elements that can be varied for good taste and versatility. First, gravies require a thickening agent such as flour, cornstarch or arrowroot. Second, they require some kind of stock seasoning such as soy sauce or vegetarian "chicken" powder. Third, they require water. Then, you can get fancy and add spices and condiments such as garlic, onions, ginger, pepper, mushrooms and other spices. To give it additional body, you can add nuts or nut butters. Just remember that if you add nut butters, they are low in EMI and such gravies must be used sparingly. The first recipe is the most basic gravy you can use. Then get creative. The other gravies are examples.

Simple Brown Gravy

- 1 C water or stock made from vegetables, seaweed or powdered seasoning
- 1/4 C whole wheat flour
- 2 to 3 Tbsp low sodium soy sauce or tamari

Place water in a pot, add soy sauce, and gradually mix in flour stirring well to break up any lumps. Heat over medium to high heat stirring constantly until well blended, then simmer for 3 to 5 minutes. Serve over grains, vegetables, potatoes, noodles or your favorite dish.

Brown Mushroom Gravy

- 2-1/2 C to 3 C water
- 1 C mushrooms, chopped
- 1/2 onion minced
- 1/2 C whole wheat pastry flour
- 2 Tbsp corn starch or arrowroot

- 1 Tbsp vegetarian "chicken" or "beef" stock powder such as "McKay's" usually found at health food stores
- 3 Tbsp low sodium soy sauce or to taste.

Heat about 1/4 cup water in a pot and saute onions and mushrooms with 1 Tbsp soy sauce until onions are translucent. Add in the flour and vegetarian powder and mix well while cooking for 3 to 4 minutes until slightly browned. Mix corn starch or arrowroot with cool water, add soy sauce and add to the mixture. Cook over medium heat and add the rest of the water while stirring to smoothen texture. Add more water if needed to thin the gravy or more flour to thicken it.

As an option, add 1 to 2 Tbsp peanut butter or other nut butter. Just be aware that nuts and nut butters are low in EMI and high in fat so use with caution.

Cashew Gravy

(Adapted from Country Life Vegetarian Cookbook, used with permission)

- 2 C hot water
- 1/2 C raw cashew pieces or whole wheat flour
- 1 Tbsp brewer's yeast
- 1 Tbsp onion powder
- 2 Tbsp whole wheat flour
- 2 Tbsp (or less) vegetarian "chicken" seasoning such as "McKay's" (or substitute)

Start with one C water in blender, add cashews, then remaining ingredients. Cook in sauce pan till thickened, stirring constantly. Use as topping for vegetables, rice or top with chopped chives or add one cup frozen peas while cooking and serve over sprouted wheat toast or baked potatoes.

Tahini Sauce

- 2 Tbsp tahini
- 2 Tbsp Tamari
- 2 Tbsp water

Place all ingredients together in a pan and cook over low flame, stirring constantly until they have blended and have the consistency of cream. Drizzle over grains.

Oriental Ginger Sauce

- 1 C water
- 2 Tbsp low-sodium soy sauce
- 1/4 tsp grated ginger
- 1 Tbsp arrowroot or cornstarch

Mix arrowroot or cornstarch in 1/4 C cool water. Add to a saucepan with the water, soy sauce and ginger. Heat at medium until thickened and stir. Serve with steamed vegetables. A fancier variation is next.

Oriental Ginger Gravy

- 2 C water
- 1/4 of an onion, minced (or 1/2 tsp onion powder)
- 2 Tbsp arrowroot
- 1-2 tsp low-sodium soy sauce or tamari to taste
- 1/2 tsp grated ginger
- 1 garlic clove (or 1/4 tsp garlic powder)

Saute the onions and garlic in a 1/4 C water in saucepan until translucent. Dissolve arrowroot in 1/4 cup of cool water. Mix all ingredients, and simmer and stir over low heat until thickened. Serve over steamed vegetables, over rice, over meat-substitutes, or even on toast or waffles.

Oriental Mushroom Gravy

- 2 C water
- 3 Tbsp soy sauce
- 2-1/2 Tbsp cornstarch or arrowroot dissolved in cool water
- 1-1/2 C finely chopped fresh mushrooms or 5 pcs
  shiitake mushrooms

If using dry mushrooms, them in warm water until rehydrated. Chop mushrooms and save the stems for stock. Use the soaking water as part of the water added to this gravy. Briefly mix water, soy sauce and cornstarch or arrowroot dissolved in cool water. Pour into saucepan and add mushrooms. Heat, stirring constantly, over medium-high until thickened. As an option, you can add chopped seitan and simmer 5 minutes so this can be used as a substitute for meat sauce. Serve over steamed vegetables, over rice, over meat-substitutes, or even on toast.

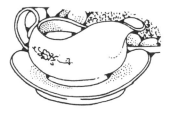

SOUPS

Corn Chowder

- 5 C Water
- 1-1/2 C corn or kernels cut from 3 ears corn
- 1 onion, diced
- 1 stalk celery, diced
- 1 clove garlic, crushed
- 1 to 2 Tbsp low-sodium soy sauce or tamari
- parsley
- (optional) 1 tsp cornstarch
- (optional) 1 Tbsp miso

If you use corn on the cob, save the cobs and simmer them for 5 - 10 minutes in water with a pinch of salt. Then saute onion, celery, and garlic in a little water and add to the corn stock. Simmer again for 10 minutes, then add corn kernels and cook 5 minutes more. Add soy sauce. For a creamy texture, take half the mixture, blend it and add back to the soup. For a thicker texture, add 1 tsp cornstarch dissolved in 2 tablespoons cold water and stir. Reheat and serve garnished with parsley. Serve whole grain crackers or rice cakes on the side.

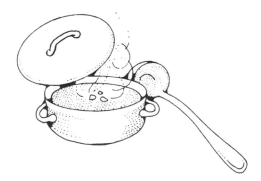

Cream of Broccoli Soup

(used by permission from Kristina Turner's Self-Healing Cookbook)

- 5 C water
- 1-1/2 C broccoli, chopped
- 1-1/2 C leftover brown rice or oatmeal
- 1 small onion, diced
- barley or white miso

Bring water or stock to a boil and add broccoli stems and onion. Cover and simmer 10 minutes. Put 2 cups of the soup liquid in the blender with rice or oatmeal. Blend until smooth, then return to the pot. Add broccoli tops and simmer until tender but still bright green. Add miso to taste by taking about 1 heaping teaspoon miso and making a puree with a little of the soup liquid. Add the puree back to the pot, warm through and serve.

MISO SOUP

Miso is a most versatile food which is made from fermented soy beans and salt. It is excellent as a no-cholesterol base for soups or for sauces. It is, however, quite high in sodium. Here are some variations of miso soup. Because miso is so flavorful, it will make almost any vegetable you put in the soup delicious.

Wakame Onion Mushroom Soup

- 1 handful wakame
- 1 onion, diced
- 4 C water from soaking the wakame
- 1 to 2 Tbsp miso
- 2 dried shiitake mushrooms

Soak wakame and mushrooms in 1 C water until soft, cut into 1-inch pieces. Saute onions in a 1/4 C water, add water from soaked wakame and mushrooms and the rest of the water, bring to a boil, add the wakame and mushrooms, and cook over low flame until it is tender. Add miso to taste by diluting 1 to 2 Tbsp miso in a ladel full of the soup water, mashing and smoothing out the miso and adding it back to the pot. Leftover grain or noodles may be added if desired.

Miso Soup with Daikon

- 1/4 C wakame
- 1 small onion, diced
- 1/2 C daikon radish, diced
- 1 handful daikon greens, chopped
- 4 C water
- 1 to 2 Tbsp miso

Place wakame, onion, and daikon in a saucepan and add water. Bring to boil, reduce flame and simmer for 20 minutes. add the greens about 5 minutes before serving so that they can remain bright green. Measure 1 to 2 Tbsp miso into a cup and add a small amount of the broth to dilute, mash and smooth out the miso. Add back to the soup and simmer for about 2 minutes.

Miso Soup Variations

Vary Miso Soup recipe using onions, cauliflower, shiitake mushrooms, celery, tofu chunks, etc. to wakame broth. May also vary by adding medium grain brown rice or barley.

Noodle Soup

This is hearty enough to be used as an entree. It is a dish that is quite easy to prepare and one that you can custom design for your taste by using any vegetables that you like.

- 1 pkg buckwheat noodles
- 1/2 onion, minced
- 1 Tbsp vegetarian "chicken" powder
- 3 - 4 Tbsp miso (to taste)
- 5 shiitake mushrooms
- 3 quarts water
- 1 thinly sliced carrot
- 1 bunch won bok cabbage
- 1 small handful dried wakame (seaweed)
- vegetables of your choice
- low-sodium soy sauce
- 3 Tbsp green onion, chopped
- black pepper

Noodle preparation: Boil a pot of water and add noodles and continue to boil. When noodles start to foam, pour in 1/2 C cool water and the foaming will stop for a while and start foaming again. Add cool water in this fashion two more times and the noodles should be done. Drain noodles in a seive or colander and rinse with cool water.

Soup preparation: Soak mushrooms in 1/4 C of water. Then place water and mushrooms in a pot and add the rest of the water. Add minced onion, dried seaweed vegetarian powder and miso that has been dissolved in a small amount of water, bring to a boil, and simmer for a few minutes. Then lighty parboil the other vegetables and place over noodles in a large bowl. Then add the soup stock over the vegetables and noodles and garnish with chopped green onion and spice with black pepper. Add low-sodium soy sauce to taste.

CLEAR SOUPS

Here are two variations of a very basic soup that are easy to prepare and that you can easily modify to your taste. The soup base is konbu seaweed and soy sauce, a delicious combination.

Clear Tamari Soup

- 6" piece of konbu
- 1/4 C daikon, sliced in thin rounds
- 2 shiitake mushrooms
- 4 C water
- low-sodium tamari or soy sauce

Rinse konbu under running water to remove excess salt. Place in saucepan, add shiitake and daikon, and water. Cover and bring to a boil, reduce flame and simmer for 20 to 30 minutes. Add 1 to 2 tablespoons tamari to the broth. Remove the shiitakes and slice thin, remove stems and return to the broth. Remove the konbu and save for cooking with beans at another time. Serve in individual bowls. Garnish with a sprig of watercress or parsley.

Clear Cauliflower Soup

- 5 C water
- 1/2 large cauliflower (cut into flowerettes)
- 6" piece konbu
- low sodium soy sauce or tamari to taste

Rinse konbu and soak in 1/4 C warm water until tender and slice into 1" pieces. In a sauce pan, place konbu, cauliflower, and water including soaking water. Bring to a boil, covered. Reduce flame and simmer until cauliflower is tender. Add soy sauce or tamari to taste.

Lentil Soup

- 1 C lentils
- 4-5 C water
- 1 medium onion
- 1 broccoli stalk, chopped
- 1 celery stalks, sliced into 1/2" pieces
- 1 carrot, sliced into thin pieces
- Sea salt or low-sodium soy sauce
- 2 bay leaves
- 2 Tbsp chopped parsley

- Optional vegetables e.g. burdock, potatoes, seaweed, daikon
- Optional seasoning, 2 tsp cumin. Vegetable, miso or powdered vegetarian "chicken" stock can be substituted for some
  of the salt or soy sauce.

Wash lentils and place in saucepan with water. Bring to a boil
and lower heat to low. Simmer 20 to 30 minutes. Add diced
onions, broccoli, celery and other vegetables, simmer until
vegetables are soft (about another 15 to 20 minutes depending
on the size of chopped vegetables. If cut in larger chunks, you
will need to add them sooner so they cook longer). Add salt or
soy sauce and other seasonings to taste.

Quick Red Lentil Soup

For a quick lentil soup, use red lentils (actually they're
orange). Follow above instructions but use red lentils and simmer for just 10 minutes.

Split Pea Soup

- 8 C water
- 2 C split peas
- 1/4 C barley
- 2 onions, chopped
- 2 stalk celery, diced
- 1 carrot, diced
- 1 tsp basil or 1/2 tsp marjoram
- 1 tsp thyme
- 2 bay leaves
- 1/4 C soy sauce or miso dissolved in hot water to taste
- Other vegetables such as parsnips, burdock or potato.

Wash split peas well and boil with barley, onions and bay leaf (and parsnips or potato, if any) in 4 C water for 30 minutes. Add other vegetables, herbs and spices, 4 C water and simmer another 30 minutes. Add soy sauce or miso to taste before serving.

FRUIT AND DESSERTS

SWEET DELIGHTS

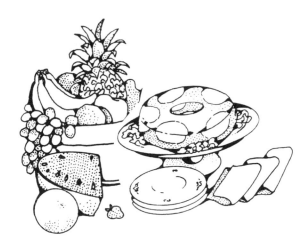

Fruits are generally good weight loss foods because most of them are high in EMI. They also contain a wealth of vitamins such as beta-carotene and vitamin C. There are some exceptions, however, including, most notably, dried fruit. It would be nice to eat fruit to our heart's content. However, the problem with fruit is it's high sugar content. Fruits contain fructose, a natural fruit sugar that can be absorbed very quickly. And although its not as bad as white sugar, it has some of the negative properties of its table-sugar cousin and does tend to cause a rise in triglycerides (storage fats) in our blood. High triglycerides are a co-risk-factor with cholesterol for heart disease.

Nonetheless, fruits are good as dessert and a way to satisfy a "sweet tooth." Some people find that fruits are easier to digest if they are cooked. Others find that they do better with raw fruit or feel that they do better if fruit is eaten by itself rather than with other foods at a meal. Still others recommend "fruit fasts" as an effective way to lose weight, and while I don't recommed this approach, the EMI explains why this actually works. My experience is that how people do with fruit varies from person to person and can change with time. If possible, try to eat fruit in season and from your locality, and remember that your main food should be grain and vegetables rather than fruit. As for prepared desserts, most of them have a lot of butter, oil, shortening, and simple sugar added so that they become quite low in EMI. For example, a whole apple is about 90 calories. A slice of apple pie can be 350 calories or nearly four times as much in calories. Instead, I like to use whole fruits as a basis of desserts. Here are a few examples of prepared dishes based on whole fruit.

Baked Apple with Raisin Sauce

• 5 Apples (Rome, Pippin, Granny Smith, or Jonathan are good
  baking apples)
• 1 C apple juice
• 1/4 C raisins
• 1 tsp cinnamon
• 1/2 tsp vanilla
• 1 Tbsp arrowroot (or cornstarch)

Preheat oven to 375 degrees. Wash apples, cut off the top and core into the apple about halfway down to get the seeds out but not to poke through the bottom. Place into a baking pan with a small amount of water and bake for 15 to 20 minutes. Place apple juice, raisins, cinnamon, vanilla, and a pinch of salt into a saucepan and bring to a boil. Then simmer at low heat for 5 minutes. Dissolve the arrowroot in cool water and add to mixture and stir. Spoon sauce into the apples and enjoy.

Natural Fruit "Gelatin"

Most people are unaware that gelatin dessert is an animal product even though they come in fruit flavors. Supermarket gelatin comes from boiling down animal tendons and hoofs for its gelatinous proteins. A better source, I believe, is the "gelatin" that comes from agar, a seaweed product. You can use any fruit in it and any fruit juice for sweetening. The agar comes in a dried bar or in the form of flakes. Here's an example.

Cantaloupe Strawberry "Gelatin"

- 1 cantaloupe
- 3 small boxes strawberries
- 6 cups water
- 2 cups apple juice
- 2 bars agar

Make cantaloupe into balls and reserve juice to add to mixture. Add water to juice. Break agar into this mixture, soak until dissolved. Bring to a boil, reduce flame, and simmer for 20 to 30 minutes. Partially chill, add cantaloupe balls and strawberries. Refrigerate and chill until completely firm.

Fruit Compote

(Contributed by Kathy Cain)

- 2 Pears (or nectarines, peaches or apples)
- 1 C apple juice (or to cover 1/2" of pan)
- 2 pinches sea salt
- 1/8 C water
- 1 tsp arrowroot
- 3 - 4 Tbsp almond slivers
- 1/2 tsp cinnamon
- 1 handful raisins
- Optional mint leaf for garnish,

Cut pears, nectarines, peaches or apples into 1" chunks. Place in a saucepan in 1/2" of apple juice, and add one pinch of sea salt per fruit. Add cinnamon and raisins if you wish. Bring to boil and simmer for 1 to 2 minutes until fruit is slightly tender but firm. Thicken the juice by adding arrowroot dissolved in 1/8 C water then simmer another minute. Serve in dish or sherbet glass sprinkled with toasted almond slivers and a mint leaf.

Chunky Apple Sauce

- 4 to 6 apples, peeled and cut into chunks
- apple juice
- 1 tsp cinnamon powder
- 4 whole allspice
- 4 whole cloves

Place sliced apples into pot. Add just enough apple juice to cover the bottom. Mix in spices and bring just to a boil. Lower the heat and simmer for 15 to 20 minutes, or until apples are soft but still with some texture. This is also good on toast or pancakes or waffles. (see section on fancy breakfasts)

Almond Milk

Remember that all nuts are low in EMI and should be used sparingly. In addition, remember that the beverage of choice is water or other non-caloric beverages.

- 1/4 C almonds
- 1 C water
- 1 apple, peeled and diced (optional)

Grind almonds fine in the blender. Then add water and optional apple and blend into a creamy milk.

Apple Crisp

- 5 Apples (Rome, Jonathan, or Granny Smith are good choices but others will do)
- 5 pinches sea salt
- 5 tsp lemon juice
- 1/4 C pastry flour
- 3 Tbsp chopped walnuts
- 1 C rolled oats
- 1 Tbs cinnamon
- sesame oil (to oil pan)
- 1/4 tsp nutmeg (optional)
- 1/4 tsp vanilla (optional)

Slice apples vertically into slivers about 1/4 inch thick. Place in oiled saucepan. Drizzle with lemon juice. Sprinkle with sea salt. Then mix the flour, oats, cinnamon, walnuts and nutmeg together and sprinkle over apples. Bake at 350 degrees for 10 minutes covered with foil and 5 minutes without cover to brown.

Carrot Cake

(Contributed by Elaine French)

- 1/2 cup grated carrot
- 1 1/4 cups chopped dates
- 1 cup raisins
- 1 1/4 cups water
- 1/2 cup unsweetened applesauce
- 1 tsp. cinnamon
- 1 tsp. allspice
- 1/2 tsp. nutmeg
- 1/4 tsp. cloves
- 2 cups whole wheat flour
- 1 tsp. baking soda
- 1 tsp. baking powder

Preheat oven to 350 degrees. Oil and flour an 8" x 8" cake pan, or use a non-stick pan. Combine carrots, dates, raisins, water, applesauce, cinnamon, allspice, nutmeg and cloves in a saucepan. Bring to a boil, reduce the heat and simmer for 5 minutes. Cool. In a separate bowl stir together the flour, baking soda and baking powder. Combine the wet and dry mixtures and stir just until mixed. Spread the batter evenly into the pan and bake for 45 to 50 minutes.

Pineapple Cheesecake

(Contributed by Elaine French)

- 1/4 cup Emes gelatin
- 1/2 cup water
- 1 1/2 cups Grapenuts cereal
- 20-ounce block firm tofu
- 1/2 cup fructose powder
- 1 tsp. lemon juice
- 1 tsp. vanilla
- 3/4 cup (6 ounce) frozen pineapple juice concentrate, thawed

In a small saucepan, combine the Emes gelatin and water and set aside to soften. Spread the Grapenuts in the bottom of a 9" x 12" pan. In a blender or food processor, combine the tofu, fructose, lemon juice, vanilla and pineapple juice concentrate. Blend until smooth.

Dissolve the gelatin in the water over low heat, add it to the tofu mixture and blend again. Place a very small bowl or cup in the center of the Grapenuts crust. Slowly pour the tofu mixture into the bowl so the mixture gently flows over the edges and on to the crust. (This will keep the Grapenuts on the bottom so they don't swirl around in the tofu mixture.) Carefully remove the cup. Smooth out the surface of the cheesecake if necessary and refrigerate for one hour to set.

You may add crushed pineapple as a topping before serving if you like.

GLOSSARY

Arame: A high-calcium food (like almost all seaweeds) and is a Japanese seaweed which appears to be another "stringy" sea vegetable like hijiki when you buy it, but it is actually a flat seaweed that is finely sliced to its stringy appearance. Because it is sliced, the cut edges are exposed and it therefore cooks slightly faster than hijiki.

Chapati: An East Indian unleavened flat bread that is much like flour tortillas.

Hijiki: A high-calcium food which is a stringy Japanese seaweed similar to arame.

Konbu: A broad, thick seaweed also known as kelp or laminaria that is used both as a high calcium food as well as the basis of soup stock.

Miso: A fermented soy paste product which has a savory flavor often used in soups and sauces.

Pita Bread: A flat round bread that when cut in two forms two pieces of pocket bread that can be stuffed to make sandwiches.

Seitan: Also known as wheat gluten which has the chewy texture of meat and is used as a meat subsitute.

Shiitake Mushroom: A delicious Japanese mushroom, sold in its dried form and easily used by soaking in water.

TVP: An abbreviation for texturized vegetable protein used for making sauses have the texture of ground meat.

Tahini: Sesame butter.

Tamari: Genuine tamari is soy sauce made naturally without wheat as a by-product of miso making. However, it is commonly used as a term simply describing naturally brewed soy sauce.

Tempeh: A whole soybean food that is a good meat substitute. It is fermented which minimizes its "beany" flavor and gassiness.

Umeboshi: A Japanese pickled plum which has a strong tart and salty flavor. In Japan it is used as a condiment as well as a folk medicine.

Wakame: A tender leafy Japanese seaweed, high in calcium as in other seaweeds.

Vegetarian "chicken" seasoning: A powdered product that is made from vegetable products and spices that has a chicken flavor. It is used for soup bases and gravies.

PART III

Stay Healthy with the
Eat More, Weigh Less Diet

CHAPTER 11

Let Food Be Your Medicine

Most of this book has been focused on how you can lose weight by eating more of the foods that promote weight loss. But the main point of the Eat More Diet is to make you healthy. In addition to helping you to improve your health, it can also drastically reduce your health care costs. This has been demonstrated repeatedly in my experience with diet and is supported by some of the latest medical literature.

GETTING RID OF TWO HEADACHES

Four years ago, in my private practice, I saw a patient named Larry who had headaches for over 20 years. He reported that he was constantly on pain medication for headaches 5 out of 7 days a week, and that it was interfering with his life. He had been hospitalized three times in the past for the headaches and had been CAT scanned twice at great expense (he estimated his total medical bills at $250,000) and to no avail. After I put him on a diet similar to the Eat More Diet, the headaches began to subside in four days and disappeared in ten days. Thereafter, he no longer needed any ongoing pain medication. The total cost for this was less than $175. Larry told me I'd gotten rid of his headache of medical and drug costs. I said what about his other headache. He said he'd already forgotten about that one, and we laughed.

HEART DISEASE

Seventy percent of all Americans die of a diet related disease according to modern statistics. The sad thing about these statistics is that most of these diseases are treatable and even curable with a dietary approach.

THE LEADING KILLER of Americans is cholesterol-related disease which includes heart disease (35.7%), strokes (7%) and other forms of atherosclerosis (1.1%). If you add these up, the number is fully 43.8 % of all of us dying in the U.S. of these diseases, a staggering 931,100 people. (1) Cholesterol kills by accumulating over the years in the blood vessels and plugging them up. If the occlusion occurs in the heart, a heart attack may occur. If it happens in the brain, a stroke occurs. Diet and blood cholesterol levels are directly related to these deaths. There is such a close relationship that for every one percent increase in cholesterol, there is a two percent increase in risk of heart attack. In fact, no one with a blood cholesterol level of 150 mg/dl or less ever died of a heart attack in the most respected nutrition and heart disease study in the world, the Framingham Study from Harvard University. (2)

LOWER YOUR CHOLESTEROL IN 21 DAYS

In 1989, I and my colleagues at the Waianae Coast Comprehensive Health Center demonstrated that cholesterol could be reduced by an average of 14% through diet alone within three weeks. (3) A number of studies indicate that diet can indeed lower cholesterol significantly and thus reduce the risk of heart disease. (4,5,6,7) In 1990, Dr. Dean Ornish of the University of San Francisco conducted a study that demonstrated that atherosclerosis could be reversed by putting patients on a diet similar to ours in fat content without medication. In that study, the disease in patients on the "control" diet which was 30% fat (which many health organizations recommend) continued to worsen. (8)

The irony is that while insurance does not pay for nutrition counseling to prevent these arteries from occlusion, or to treat them with nutrition after they get become occluded, they will pay $25,000 to $100,000 for coronary bypass surgery. This will be done despite large studies which indicate that surgery does not prolong life in most of the cases and have found "[no] significant overall risk reduction with surgery." (9) Aside from the specific instances in which benefit is clear, (left main artery disease, for example), the usual indication is unmanageable chest pain. However, chest pain is also manageable through a good diet (10,11,12). Moreover, the person who has

Cholesterol and Heart Disease
Heart Attack vs Serum Cholesterol

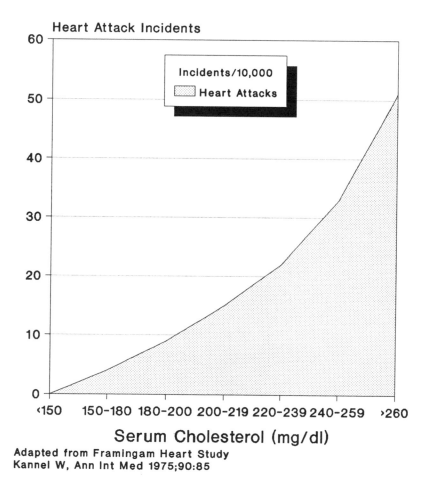

Adapted from Framingam Heart Study
Kannel W, Ann Int Med 1975;90:85

undergone the bypass needs to be on a therapeutic diet anyway or the bypass and other arteries will become occluded at roughly the same rate as it would have without the bypass. (13,14)

SIX STEPS TO LOWERING CHOLESTEROL

1. Avoid or limit Cholesterol Intake
2. Avoid or limit Fat Intake
3. Eat More High EMI Foods
4. Avoid or limit Saturated Fat Intake
5. Avoid or limit Coffee and Smoking
6. Exercise

HIGH BLOOD PRESSURE

Using a similar dietary approach, even some of the highest blood pressures I have treated respond to special diets even without medication. The validity of such an approach is supported by our research and that of other researchers. (15,16).

YOUR BEST DEFENSE AGAINST CANCER

Cancer now afflicts one in three Americans. Nearly 22% of all Americans eventually die of cancer at today's rates and despite all our efforts, cancer deaths are on the rise. When I first started studying the relationship between diet and cancer in the mid-seventies, it was considered on the "fringe" of medicine. Today, the National Cancer Institute considers diet to be the #1 cause of cancer.

CAUSES OF CANCER

Diet 35%
Smoking 30%
Genetic 15%
Environmental 10%
Other 10%

In fact, some researchers believe that up to 70% of all cancers are diet-related.

Support for this view comes from studies that relate the following dietary factors to certain cancers

Low Fiber –
Colon Cancer

High Fat –
Breast Cancer
Colon Cancer
Prostate Cancer

High Animal Protein –
Breast Cancer
Prostate Cancer

Low Beta Carotene –
Lung Cancer
Breast Cancer
Prostate Cancer
Stomach Cancer
Esophageal Cancer

Recent research has uncovered many items as "anti-oxidants" that can help prevent the early stages of cancer. These studies suggest that anti-oxidants such as vitamin C, Vitamin E, beta carotene, and selenium help to neutralize substances that could cause the "oxidation" of the cell's DNA and create mutations that could turn a good cell into a cancerous one.

Diet can be important in both the prevention and the treatment of cancer. A healthy bodily system is important in warding off cancers and in battling cancer in those who have been found to have cancer. Just be sure that a dietary approach is not a substitute for professional care by a medical doctor.

DIABETES

Diabetes among all the chronic diseases is one where some emphasis has been placed on diet. Diabetes has even been nicknamed by lay people "sugar diabetes" because high blood sugar is the hallmark of the disease. The American Diabetes Association has a diet plan which is commonly known as an

DIETARY FAT AND DIABETES
Effect of dietary fat on
glucose tolerance

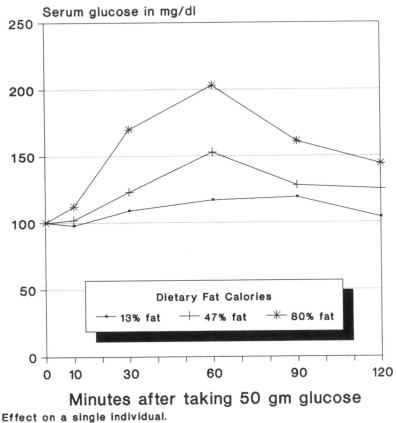

Serum glucose in mg/dl

Minutes after taking 50 gm glucose

Effect on a single individual.
Himsworth HP, Clin Sci, 1935;2:67-94.

"ADA diet". While such a diet helps many people, there is some debate going on at this time as to whether other approaches are useful. For example there are studies that show that a high complex carbohydrate, high fiber, very low fat diet can control and even reverse diabetes. (3,15,16,17) There is also evidence that certain foods seem to "protect" against diabetes. (18)

With the dietary approach described in this book, many patients have been able to reduce their requirement for some or all diabetes medication through diet. While the effect of this approach varies from individual to individual, the ability of at least some patients to reduce their medication was confirmed in the Waianae Diet Program which we conducted in Hawaii. (3) Some patients have been taken off as much as 60 units of insulin through diet alone, and kept off for years with normal or near normal blood sugars. If you have diabetes and/or are taking medication for diabetes, do not attempt this without medical supervision. Check with your medical doctor before making any changes in your diet.

ARTHRITIS

The Arthritis Foundation points out that there is no diet for arthritis. However, there is a growing body of evidence that arthritis can be improved in some patients by a good diet. In October 1991, a physician named Jenis Kjeld-Kragh reported (19) that arthritis improved after a special diet coupled with an initial period of fasting. Other researchers have demonstrated similar results. (20,21) These studies reflect the experience I have had with patients with rheumatoid arthritis as well as osteoarthritis.

OTHER ILLNESSES

There is no room to list all the diseases treatable through nutrition. Some of the others include acne, constipation, gastritis, peptic ulcer disease, fatigue, PMS, obesity, rash, and many others. While the literature supporting the therapeutic value of diet on some of these illnesses varies in strength, in any case, one should consider diet as an alternative. After all, for the average adult, following a diet of whole food is essentially harmless and the only side effects are good side effects such as weight loss and decreased cholesterol. This is more that you can say for any medications.

Thomas Edison once said:

"The doctor of the future will give
no medicine, but will interest his patient ... in diet and in
the cause and prevention of disease."

And Hippocrates said:
"Let food be thy medicine."

CHAPTER 12

Eat More and Weigh Less
The Rest of Your Life

I hope you've had fun reading this book and trying out the Eat More diet. I also hope you've learned something interesting about food such as, how it requires 30 ears of corn or 31 apples to make one day's worth of calories. With the Eat More Index, you've learned how it takes 4.6 pounds of brown rice, 9.6 pounds of potatoes, 13 pounds of carrots, 27.3 pound of grapefruit or 39 pounds of chinese cabbage to provide one day's worth of calories. You have the Eat More Index that can give you this information and help you select the foods that can fill you up, make you satisfied, and allow you to eat as much as you want. Now that you are armed with this information, you have greater control of your weight and even more importantly, your health. The challenge as with any diet is to now make it part of your life and to sustain these dietary changes for good.

The reason I tried to make this book as interesting and enjoyable as possible is that we tend to remember and act on things that are appealing and interesting. The following four step summary is included here to help you maintain the Eat More Diet.

STEP 1: ENJOY VARIETY IN YOUR DIET

Variety is the spice of life. And with food, spice is the key to variety. I encourage you to spice up your foods just the way you like them. Discover how to use spices, herbs and other non-fat flavorings to add zest and taste to everything you eat. The recipes in this book are just a start. Using the Eat More Diet concept, the EMI and the "Inverted Pyramid," I hope you will learn to create more and more enjoyable variety in your meals.

Most people in America use only three tastes over and over: grease, salt and sugar. How boring and how unhealthy can we be. With the Eat More Diet, I encourage you to eat a greater variety of foods and to flavor it with a greater variety of spices. You will be pleasantly surprised at the delicious foods that will become your favorite foods. When you eliminate the overpowering flavor of grease, excess salt, and excess sugar, you will begin to enjoy the subtle tastes of foods that you never recognized before. And when you begin to enjoy these flavors, you will want to continue this way of eating for the rest of your life.

STEP 2: HAVE A POSITIVE ATTITUDE

One of the most effective elements of the Eat More Diet program is that it has a built-in psychological mechanism for keeping you on the program. The EMI of Food helps you look at foods in a totally different light—from a positive perspective rather than a negative one. It allows you to see food from a perspective of abundance rather than deprivation. I can't point out too often that almost all other diets emphasize deprivation—"don't eat this, don't eat that." They begin from the point of psychological negativity, so it's small wonder that the results are also negative. The Eat More Diet helps to address this problem from the positive perspective, by emphasizing foods that help you lose weight.

Let me give you an example of how this works. In general the human mind is a wonderful mechanism and tends to move the individual toward mental pictures. If a person pictures in their mind a goal, then the mind will direct the person consciously or subconsciously to move toward that goal. In the same way, if you tell a people not to eat fried bacon, and give them no other image, the mind may cause them to crave and move toward eating bacon. It's like telling someone not to think of pink elephants.

TRY NOT TO THINK OF PINK ELEPHANTS

Try it yourself. Try not to think of pink elephants. Give it your best effort - and be honest. Give it a little time - try not thinking about a line of pink elephants with their trunks holding the tails of the others. Try not thinking about the last pink elephant that is the cute little baby elephant. I'm sure you'll see that you can't not think of the pink elephants, right? Now try not thinking of fried bacon... about three slices of sizzling bacon bubbling in its grease and the smell wafting through the room. Try as hard as you can for a moment. Can't do it can you? Now try not thinking about a blue forest. Try as hard as you can now. Don't think about the wonder of blue leaves and purple tree trunks. Forget about the brilliant orange birds chirping in the branches of the trees as the contrast against the background of the blue forest. Again, you can't not think of a blue forest. But wait—! You no doubt noticed that for that instant, the instant that you were trying not to see the blue forest, you were not thinking of pink elephants—were you? And, for that matter you weren't thinking of fried bacon either.

In the same way, having you concentrate on what foods to eat such as savory wild rice, or pasta primavera is much more effective—at least for most individuals— because the emphasis is on what to eat instead of on what not to eat. The EMI helps you focus on the positive aspects of eating. It is based more on the weight of the food you should eat rather than the calories you should not. It helps to plant the image of what to do to lose weight in your mind instead of the negative things that cause you to gain weight. In this way, the Eat More Diet Program provides a positive image of what you should be eating for the rest of your life.

STEP 3: PLAY YOUR FAT AWAY

Don't forget that play should be exercise and exercise should be play. Remember the good feeling you've had when you were a child running around playing tag. Remember that your body produces its own substances that make you feel so good that that if you do it often enough, you'll get hooked on it. Perhaps the most important thing about play is that if you play regularly, that is 4 times a week at least 30 to 40 minutes, it helps you lose weight while you sleep. If you think you are too busy, let me assure you that exercising regularly will give you more energy than you thought you ever could have. You'll then find that you'll actually have more time on your hands because you'll get more done in a shorter period of time and enjoy it more. Try it and see.

STEP 4: SHARE THE CONCEPT WITH OTHERS

Lack of social support system is another reason diets fail today. It can be difficult sustaining an eating pattern that is different from the people around you. This is why one of the most important thing you can do to stay on the program is sharing the Eat More Diet with others. You not only help them but you also help yourself by tapping their energy and boosting your own to stay on the program. My most successful patients are those whose spouses and families go on the program together.

Mr. Boyer is a good example. It was easy for him to stay on the diet because his wife was very enthusiastic about the program. They shopped, cooked and ate the Eat More Diet way and lost weight together. She hounded him at first but after a few weeks, he began to truly enjoy and crave the food. In fact he can't understand why he liked the food he used to eat. "It's too salty now," he says about his old Standard American Diet (notice the very appropriate acronym, SAD). And after he saw his 31-pound weight loss in 3 months, he couldn't complain. His wife lost only 4 pounds but at 5'3" tall and 123 pounds, she had little weight to lose to begin with.

But sharing in small family groups or with friends is only part of the importance of social support. The other important element is the impact your actions have to "secular trends"— in other words, how the rest of society is moving. In the secular trends in the way people eat, there have been some positive changes in these past fifteen or so years. Dietary fat has decreased from 42 percent to 38 percent in the American diet. In recent years, deaths from heart disease have also decreased from 49 percent down to 35 percent. You can help save many people in this country by contributing to this wonderful secular trend towards a healthy America and an healthy world. Excitement is contagious. Once you see what the Eat More Diet can do for you, share this excitement with a friend. This helps increase the number of people eating this way and help move the secular trends toward eating better. It will also increase the amount of positive feed-back you'll get from your peers, who may join you on the diet and may therefore help you stick with the program even while they're helping themselves. There's something inherently nice about positive things — they're contagious!

IMPRESS YOUR FRIENDS WITH THE EAT MORE DIET

One way to begin this ripple effect is to share some of the startling facts you'll learn in this book with others. Discuss them. Don't be surprised if people are surprised and even argumentative when you first tell them that the best way to lose weight is to eat more. Just learn the simple principles so you can explain them to others, show them the EMI table and tell them some of the startling poundages of food it requires to make one-day's calories (e.g. 9.6 pounds of potatoes!). Also show them the picture in this book about how you can eat nearly three times as much while eating fewer calories. Then try the "impress your friends lunch" described in chapter 9. Doing this will also help encourage you to integrate the program into your own lifestyle, for the better you understand what you're doing, the more confident you'll be.

DO IT FOR YOU!

This diet program may literally change your life so stick with the program for at least 14 days and preferably 30 days. It may be difficult at first eating all that food, but believe me, the rewards are worth the adjustment. If you are overweight, you'll lose weight automatically. You'll likely feel even better than you ever have in the past. You may even get rid of your need for some medications with your doctor's guidance. Remember that with the Eat More Diet, you can help yourself avoid six of the ten leading causes of death in America. Remember the simple principles of this program and how you can Eat More and Weigh Less. Remember that you are a very important person. Remember to do it for you.

BIBLIOGRAPHY

Introduction

1. Foster WR, Burton BT. "Health Implications of Obesity. NIH Consensus Development Conference. Introduction." Ann Internal Med, 1985;103:981-982.

2. Pamuck ER, "Long-term benefits and adverse effects of weight loss: weight loss and mortality in a national cohort of adults 1971 - 1987. Methods for Voluntary Weight Loss and Control: NIH Technology Assessment Conference March 30 - April 1, 1992, 148.

3. Shintani TT, Hughes CK, Beckham S, O'Connor HK. Obesity and cardiovascular risk intervention through ad-libitum feeding of traditional Hawaiian diet. Am J Clin Nutr, 1991;53:1647S.

4. U.S. Department of Health and Human Services. THE SURGEON GENERAL'S REPORT ON NUTRITION AND HEALTH, Warner Books, Inc., New York, NY 1989.

5. Burton BT, Boster WR, et al. Health implications of obesity: an NIH consensus development statement conference. Int J of Obesity. 1985;9:155-69.

6. Higgins M et al. Hazards of Obesity: The Framingham Experience, Acta Medica Scand, Suppl. 1987;723:23-36.

7. Simopoulos AP, Van Itallie TB. Body weight, health and longevity, Ann Internal Med, 1984;100:285-95.

Chapter 1

1. National Research Council. Diet and Health: Implications For Reducing Chronic Disease Risk. Washington, D.C.: National Academy Press, 1989.

2. National Center for Health Statistics. Health, United States, 1987. D.H.H.S, pub. no. (PHS) 88-1232. Public Health Service. Washington. U.S. Government Printing Office, March, 1988.

3. Whittemore AS, Wu-Williams AH, Lee M, et al. Diet physical activity, and colorectal cancer among Chinese in North America and China. JNCI, 1990;82;11:915-26.

4. Romieu I, Willett, WC, Stampfer, MJ, et al. Energy intake and other determinants of relative weight. Am J Clin Nutr 1988;47:406-12.

Chapter 2

1. Massey JT, Parsons VL, Tadros W. Design and estimation for the National Health Interview Survey 1985-94. National Center for Health Statistics, 1989; DHHS publication no. (PHS) 89-1384. (Data evaluation and methods research: series 2, no. 110).

2. Wynden R. Memorandum on Federal Government's ability to oversee $33 billion diet business. Washington, DD: House of Representatives, Committee on Small Business, Subcommittee on Regulation, Business Opportunities, and Energy, March 1990.

3. U.S. Weight Loss and Diet Control Market. Lynbrook, New York: Market Data Enterprises.

4. Ravussin E, et al. Energy Expenditure Before and During Restriction in Obese Patients, Am J Clin Nutr, 1985;41:753-759.

5. Brownell KD et al. The Effects of Repeated Cycles of Weight Loss and Regain in Rats, Physiol and Behav, 1986;38(4):459-64.

6. Council on Foods and Nutrition, A critique of low-carbo-hydrate ketogenic weight reducition regimens: A review of Dr. Atkins' diet revolution. JAMA, 1973;224(10):1415.

7. Acheson KJ, Schutz Y, Bessard T, et al. Glycogen storage capacity and de novo lipogenesis during massive carbohy-drate overfeeding in man. Am J Clin Nutr 1988;48:240-7.

8. Acheson KJ, Schutz Y, Bessard T, et al. Nutritional influences on lipogenesis and thermogenesis after a   car-bohydrate meal. Am J Physiol 1984;246 (Endocrinol Metab 9): E62-E70.

Chapter 3

1. Morley JE, Levine AS, Appetite Regulation, Postgrad Med 1985;77:42-54.

2. Welsh SO, Marston RM, Review of trends in food use in the United States, 1909 to 1980. J Am Dietetic Assn 1982;81:121-5.

3. Shintani TT, Hughes CK, Beckham S, O'Connor HK. Obesity and cardiovascular risk intervention through ad-libitum feeding of traditional Hawaiian diet. Am J Clin Nutr, 1991;53:1647S.

4. Duncan KH, Bacon JA, Weinsier RL. The effects of high and low energy density diets on satiety, energy intake, and eating time of obese and nonobese subjects. Am J Clin Nutr, 1983;37: 763-767.

5. Weinsier RL, Johnston MH, Doleys DM, Bacon JA. Dietary   management of obesity: evaluation of the time-energy   displacement diet in terms of its efficacy and nutritional adequacy for long-term weight control. Br J Nutr, 1982;47: 367-379.

6. Weinsier RL, Bacon JA, Birch R. Time-calorie displace-ment diet for weight control: A prospective evaluation of its adequacy for maintaining normal nutritional status. Int J Obes 1983;7:538-48.

7. Grimes DS, Gordon C. Satiety value of wholemeal and white bread. Lancet July 8, 1978;106

8. Haber GB, Heaton KW, et al. Depletion and disruption of dietary fibre: effects on satiety, plasma-glucose, and serum-insulin. Lancet Oct 1,1977:679-682.

Chapter 4

1. Donato K. Efficiency in utilization of various energy sources for growth. Am J Clin Nutr 1978;5:164-7.

2. Salmon DMW, & Flatt JP, Effect of dietary fat content on the incidence of obesity among ad libitum fed mice. Intl J Obesity 1985;9:443-449.

3. Trowell H, Burkitt, D eds. Western Diseases: Their emergence and prevention. Harvard University Press, Cambridge MA, 1981.

4. Young TK, Sevenhuysen G. Obesity in northern Canadian Indians: patterns, determinants, and consequences. Am J Clin Nutr 1989;49:786-93.

5. West KM. Diabetes in American Indians and other native populations of the New World. Diabetes 1974;23:841-855.

6. Taylor RJ, Zimmet PZ. Obesity and diabetes in Western Samoa. International Journal of Obesity 1981;5:367-376.

7. Romieu I, Willett, WC, Stampfer, MJ, et al. Energy intake and other determinants of relative weight. Am J Clin Nutr 1988;47:406-12.

8. Acheson KJ, Schutz Y, Bessard T, et al. Glycogen storage capacity and de novo lipogenesis during massive carbohydrate overfeeding in man. Am J Clin Nutr 1988;48:240-7.

9. Acheson KJ, Schutz Y, Bessard T, et al. Nutritional influences on lipogenesis and thermogenesis after a carbohydrate meal. Am J Physiol 1984, 246 (Endocrinol. Metab. 9): E62-E70.

10. Flatt JP, Ravussin E, Acheson KJ et al. Effects of dietary fat on post prandial substrate oxidation and on carbohydrate and fat balances. J Clin Investig 76;1019-24, 1985.

11. Dreon DM, Frey-Hewitt B, Ellsworth N, et al. Dietary fat: carbohydrate ratio and obesity in middle-aged men. Am J Clin Nutr 1988;47:995-1000.

12. Shintani TT, Hughes CK, Beckham S, O'Connor HK. Obesity and cardiovascular risk intervention through ad-libitum feeding of traditional Hawaiian diet. Am J Clin Nutr, 1991;53:1647S.

13. Buzzard IM, Asp EH, Chlebowski RT, et al. Diet intervention methods to reduce fat intake: Nutrient and food group composition of self-selected low-fat diets. J Am Dietetic Assn 1990;90(1):42-53.

14. Lissner LL, Strupp DA, Kawlwarf HJ, et al. Dietary fat intake and the regulation of energy intake in human subjects. Am J Clin Nutr. 1987;46:886-92.

15. Kendall A, Levitsky DA, Strupp BJ, et al. Weight loss on a low-fat diet: consequence of the imprecision of the control of food intake in humans. Am J Clin Nutr 1991;53:1124-9.

Chapter 5

1. Bogardus C, et al. Familial Dependence of the Resting Metabolic Rate. New Engl J Med, 1986;315(2):96-100.

2. Fontaine E, et al. Resting Metabolic Rate in Monozygotic and Dizygotic Twins. Acta Genet Med Gemellol 1985;43:41-7.

3. Hurni M, Burnand B, et al. Metabolic effects of a mixed and a high-carbohydrate low-fat diet in man, measured over 24 h in a respiration chamber. Br J Nutr 1982;47:33-41.

4. Simopoulos AP. Diet, exercise, and calorie balance, JAMA 1988;260(13):1953.

5. McArdle WD, Toner M. "Application of Exercise for Weight Control: The Exercise Prescription," In: Frankle, RT and Yang, MU eds. <u>Obesity and Weight Control: The Health Professional's Guide to Understanding and Treatment</u>, Aspen Publishers, Inc., Rockville, Maryland, 254-274, 1988.

6. Lennon D, et al. Diet and exercise training effects on resting metabolic rate. Int J of Obesity 1985 39-47

7. Pi-Sunyer FX. "Exercise in the Treatment of Obesity," In: Frankle, R.T. and Yang, M.U.(eds.), <u>Obesity and Weight control: The Health Professional's Guide to Understanding and Treatment</u>, Aspen Publishers, Inc., Rockville, Maryland, 241-255, 1988.

8. Hill JO, et al. Effects of Exercise and Food Restriction on Body Composition and Metabolic Rate in Obese Women. Am J Clin Nutr 1987;46:622-30.

9. Henson LC, et al. Effects of Exercise Training on Resting Energy Expenditure During Caloric Restriction. Am J Clin Nutr 1987;46:893-899.

Chapter 6

1. Shintani TT, Hughes CK, Beckham S, O'Connor HK. Obesity and cardiovascular risk intervention through ad-libitum feeding of traditional Hawaiian diet. Am J Clin Nutr, 1991;53:1647S.

2. Duncan KH, Bacon JA, Weinsier RL. The effects of high and low energy density diets on satiety, energy intake, and eating time of obese and nonobese subjects. Am J Clin Nutr, 1983,37, 763-767.

Food values calculated from
U.S. Department of Agriculture. Nutritive Value of Foods, USDA Home and Garden Bulletin 72 1981, and computer software "Nutritionist III", N-Squared Computing Salem Oregon.

Chapter 7

1. U.S. Department of Agriculture. Human nutrition information service, USDA Home and Garden Bulletin 252, 1992. Hyattsville MD. 1992.

2. Snowdon DA, Animal product consumption and mortality because of all causes combined, coronary heart disease, stroke, diabetes, and cancer in Seventh-day Adventists. Am J Clin Nutr, 1988;48:739-48.

3. Mazess RB, Mather W. Bone mineral content of North Alaskan Eskimos. Am J Clin Nutr 1974;27:916-25.

4. Heaney RP, et al. Calcium nutrition and bone health in the elderly. Am J Clin Nutr 1982;36:1001.

5. Dahl Jorgensen K, Joner C, Hanssen K. Relationship between cows' milk consumption and incidence of insulin dependent diabetes mellitus in childhood. Diabetes Care 1991;14(11):1001-3.

6. American Academy of Pediatrics Committee on Nutrition: The use of whole cow's milk in infancy. Pediatrics 1992;89(6pt1): P1105-9.

7. Whittemore AS, Wu-Williams AH, Lee M, et al. Diet physical activity, and colorectal cancer among Chinese in North America and China. JNCI, 1990;82;11:915-26.

8. Emerentia CH, van Berenstein J, Brussaard JH, van Schaik M. Relationship between the calcium-to-protein ratio in milk and the urinary calcium excretion in healthy adults - a controlled crossover study, Am J Clin Nutr 1990;52:142.

9. Calkins BM DHSc Executive summary of the congress. Am J Clin Nutr 1988;48:709-11.

10. Keys A. Ten Heart Attacks in U.S. for One in Japan, American Heart, 16, 1966.

11. Dwyer JT. Health aspects of vegetarian diets. Am J Clin Nutr 1988;48:712-38.

12. Kempner W, Newborg BD, Peschel RL, & Skyler JS. Treatment of massive obesity with rice/reduction diet program. Arch Int Med 1975;135:1575.

Chapter 8

1. Cooper JN, Robeck IR. Management of obesity, Virginia Med, July 1984;111:384.

2. Havlik RJ, Hubert HB, et al. Weight and hypertension. Ann Internal Med. 1983;98(pt 2):855-9.

3. Build and Blood Pressure Study, (1959): Vol 1. Chicago: Society of Actuaries.

4. Build Study, 1979 (1980): Chicago: Society of Actuaries and Association of Life Insurance Medical Directors.

5. Metropolitan Life Foundation (1983): Height and Weight Tables. New York: Metropolitan Life Insurance Co. (New York).

6. Atkinson RL, Setting Standards for Success, Methods for Voluntary Weight Loss and Control. NIH, Bethesda, MD, 58, 1992.

Chapter 9

1. Robbins J, DIET FOR A NEW AMERICA, Stillpoint Publishing, Walpole NH 1987.

2. McDougall JA, McDOUGALL'S MEDICINE: A Challenging Second Opinion, New Century Publishers, Inc. Piscataway, NJ 08854, 1985.

Chapter 10

1. Turner K. THE SELF HEALING COOKBOOK. Earthtones Press, Vashon Island, WA 1987.

2. McDougall M, THE McDOUGALL HEALTH-SUPPORT-ING COOKBOOK. New Century Publishers, Inc. Piscataway, NJ, 08854, 1986.

3. Thrash AM, EAT FOR STRENGTH. New Lifestyle Books, Seale, AL 1978.

Chapter 11

1. Surgeon General's Report on Nutrition and Health, U.S. Dept of Health and Human Services, Warner Books, New York, NY, 1989.

2. Kannel WB, Castelli WP, Gordon T. Cholesterol in the prediction of atherosclerodic disease. New perspectives based on the Framingham Study. Ann Internal Med 1979;90:85.

3. Shintani TT, Hughes CK, Beckham S, O'Connor HK. Obesity and cardiovascular risk intervention through ad-libitum feeding of traditional Hawaiian diet. Am J Clin Nutr 1991;53:1647S 1991.

4. McMurry MP, Connor WE, Cerqueira MT. Dietary choles-terol and the plasma lipids and lipoproteins in the Tarahumara Indians: a people habituated to a low choles-terol diet after weaning. Am J Clin Nutr 1982;35:741-4.

5. Sacks FM, Castelli WP, Donner A, Kass EH. Plasma lipids and lipoproteins in vegetarians and controls. New Engl J Med 1975;292:1148-55.

6. Connor WE, Connor SL. The dietary treatment of hyper-lipidemia: rationale, technique, and efficacy. Med Clin North Am 1982;66:485-518.

7. Chima CS, Miller-Kovach K, et al. Lipid management clinic: Dietary intervention for patients with hypercholesterolemia. J Am Dietetic Assn 1990;90:272-74.

8. Ornish D, Brown S, Scherwitz LW, et al. Can lifestyle changes reverse coronary heart disease? The Lifestyle Heart Trial. Lancet 1990;336:129.

9. Detre K, Murphy M, Hammermeister KE, et al. Veterans' Administration cooperative stydy of medical versus surgical treatment for stable angina. Progress report. Section 9. Effect of medical versus surgical treatment on resting left ventricular ejection fraction at five years. Prog Cardiovasc Dis, 1986;28:387.

10. Ribeiro J. The effectiveness of a low lipid diet and exercise in the management of coronary artery disease. Clinical investigations. Am Heart J 1984;108:1183.

11. Ellis F. Angina and vegan diet. Am Heart J 1977;93:803.

12. Cashin W, Sanmarco MF, Nessim SA, et al. Accellerated progression of atherosclerosis in coronary vessels with minimal lesions that are bypassed. N Engl J Med 1984;311:824.

13. Campeau L, Lesperanc J, Hermann J, et al. Loss of the improvement of angina between 1 and 7 years after aorto-coronary bypass surgery: correlations with changes in vein grafts and in coronary arteries. Circulation, 1979;60(supp): 1-5.

14. Lindahl O, Lindwall L, Spangberg A, et al. A vegan regimen with reduced medication in the treatment of hypertension. Br J Nutr. 1984;52:11.

15. Anderson JW. Hypolipidemic effects of high-carbohydrate high-fiber diets. Metabolism 1980;29:551-558.

16. Kiehm TG, Anderson JW, Ward K, Beneficial effects of a high carbohydrate, high fiber diet on hyperglycemic diabetic men. Am J Clin Nutr. 1976;29:895.

17. Himsworth HP, The dietetic factor determining the glucose tolerance and sensitivity to insulin of healthy men. Clin Sci 1935;2:67-94

18. Jenkins DJA, et al. Low glycemic index starchy foods in the diabetic diet. Am J Clin Nutr, 1988;48:248.

19. Kjeld-Kragh J, Hangen M, Borchgrevink C, et al. Controlled trial of fasting and one-year vegetarian diet in rheumatoid arthritis. Lancet 1990;338:899.

20. Hafstrom I, Ringertz B, Gyllenhammer H. Effects of fasting on disease activity, neutrophil function, fatty acid compsition, and leukotriene biosynthesis in patients with rheumatoid arthritis. Arthritis Rheum, 1988;31:585.

21. Panush R. Nutritional therapy for rheumatic diseases. Ann Intern Med 1987;106;619.

APPENDIX I
THE EAT MORE INDEX

Black bars represent the EMI value which is based on the number of pounds of food required to provide 2500 calories. Foods with an EMI value greater than 4.1 tend to promote weight loss. The higher the number, the greater the tendency to promote weight loss provided the fat content is low.

White bars represent percent fat by calories.

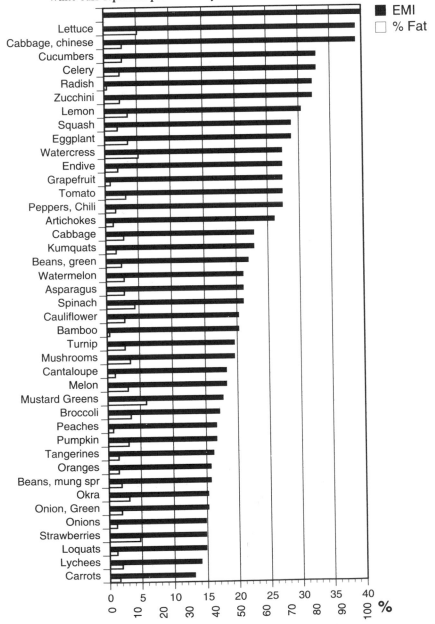

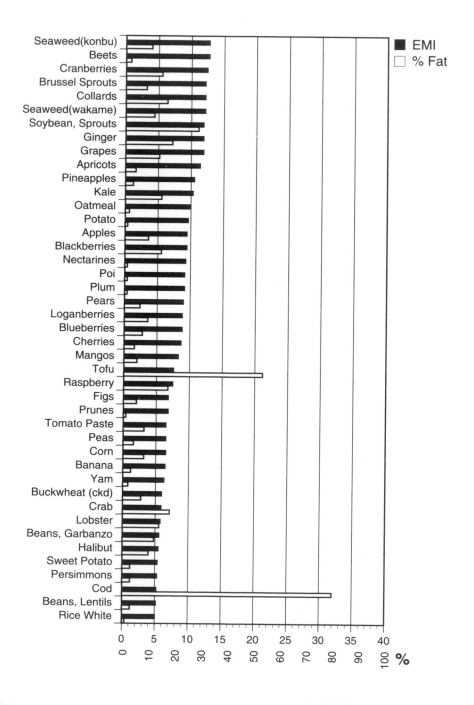

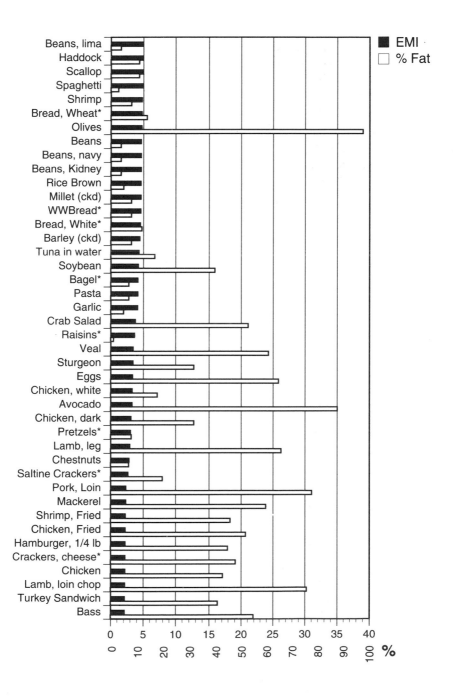

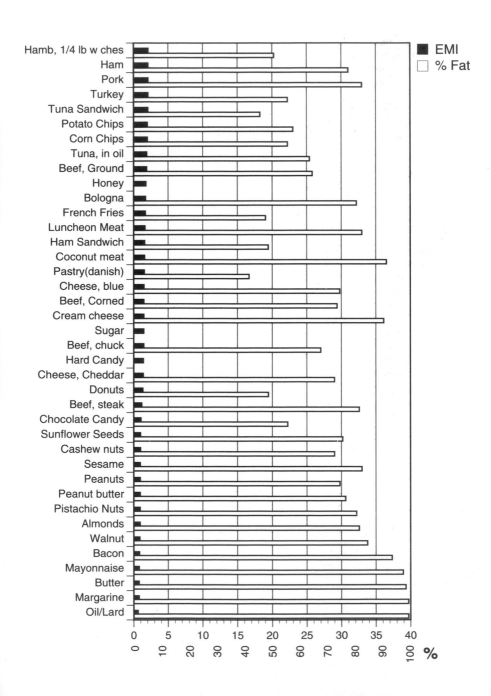

APPENDIX II
The Eat More Index (EMI) Table

The Eat More Index is based on the number of pounds of food it takes to provide 2500 calories. Percent fat by calories are also listed.

FOOD	EMI	FAT%
Almonds	0.91	82
Apples	9.42	9
Apricots	11.38	4
Artichokes	26.02	3
Asparagus	21.01	7
Avocado	3.27	88
Bacon	0.82	94
Bagel*	4.14	7
Bamboo shoots	20.23	1
Banana	6.43	3
Barley	4.43	8
Bass	2.11	55
Beans	4.63	4
Beans, garbanzo	5.58	12
Beans, green	21.85	6
Beans, kidney	4.63	4
Beans, lentils	5.15	3
Beans, lima	4.92	4
Beans, mung sprouts	15.61	5
Beans, navy	4.63	4
Beef, chuck	1.45	68
Beef, corned	1.47	74
Beef, ground	1.88	65
Beef, steak	1.16	82
Beets	12.71	2
Blackberries	9.42	14
Blueberries	8.81	7
Bologna	1.72	81
Bread, Whole Wheat*	4.73	14
Bread, White*	4.50	12
Broccoli	17.07	9
Brussels sprouts	12.14	8
Buckwheat	5.94	7

* EMI adjusted upward to account for the increase in bulk of this food in the stomach due to absorption of water

The Eat More Index (EMI) Table

The Eat More Index is based on the number of pounds of food it takes to provide 2500 calories. Percent fat by calories are also listed.

FOOD	EMI	FAT%
Butter	0.76	99
Cabbage	22.76	7
Cabbage, chinese	39.02	7
Cantaloupe	18.21	3
Carrots	13.01	4
Cashew nuts	0.97	73
Cauliflower	20.23	7
Celery	32.78	6
Cheese, blue	1.48	75
Cheese, cheddar	1.37	73
Cherries	8.67	4
Chestnuts	2.82	7
Chicken	2.19	43
Chicken, dark	3.10	32
Chicken, Fried	2.23	52
Chicken, white	3.29	18
Chocolate candy	1.04	56
Coconut meat	1.58	92
Cod	5.20	80
Collards	12.14	16
Corn	6.50	8
Corn chips	1.99	56
Crab	5.87	18
Crab salad	3.77	53
Crackers, cheese*	2.20	48
Cranberries	12.42	14
Cream cheese	1.46	91
Cucumbers	32.78	7
Donuts	1.31	49
Eggplant	28.75	9
Eggs	3.35	65
Endive	27.32	5
Figs	6.83	5

* EMI adjusted upward to account for the increase in bulk of this food in the stomach due to absorption of water

The Eat More Index (EMI) Table

The Eat More Index is based on the number of pounds of food it takes to provide 2500 calories. Percent fat by calories are also listed.

FOOD	EMI	FAT%
French fries	1.69	48
Garlic	4.11	5
Ginger	11.88	18
Grapefruit	27.32	2
Grapes	11.88	13
Haddock	4.89	11
Halibut	5.48	10
Ham	2.09	78
Ham sandwich	1.58	49
Hamb, 1/4 lb w chs	2.10	51
Hamburger, 1/4 lb	2.22	45
Hard candy	1.39	0
Honey	1.77	0
Kale	10.31	14
Kumquats	22.76	4
Lamb, leg	2.94	66
Lamb, loin chop	2.17	76
Lemon	30.35	9
Lettuce	39.02	13
Lobster	5.75	14
Loganberries	8.81	9
Loquats	14.77	3
Luncheon meat	1.64	83
Lychees	14.01	5
Mackerel	2.31	60
Mangos	8.28	5
Margarine	0.76	100
Mayonnaise	0.77	98
Melon	18.21	8
Millet	4.59	8
Mushrooms	19.51	9
Mustard greens	17.62	15
Nectarines	9.26	1

The Eat More Index (EMI) Table

The Eat More Index is based on the number of pounds of food it takes to provide 2500 calories. Percent fat by calories are also listed.

FOOD	EMI	FAT%
Oatmeal	9.93	1.6
Oil/Lard	0.61	100
Okra	15.18	8
Olives	4.71	98
Onion, green	15.18	5
Onions	14.77	3
Oranges	15.61	4
Pasta	4.14	7
Pastry(danish)	1.53	42
Peaches	16.56	2
Peanut butter	0.93	77
Peanuts	0.94	75
Pears	8.96	6
Peas	6.50	4
Peppers, chili	27.32	4
Persimmons	5.30	3
Pineapples	10.51	3
Pistachio nuts	0.92	81
Plum	9.11	1
Poi	9.11	1
Pork	2.09	83
Pork, loin	2.32	78
Potato	9.58	1
Potato chips	1.99	58
Pretzels*	3.03	8
Prunes	6.83	1
Pumpkin	16.56	8
Radish	32.14	1
Raisins*	3.64	1
Raspberry	7.48	17
Rice, brown	4.59	5
Rice, white	5.01	1
Saltine crackers*	2.64	20

* EMI adjusted upward to account for the increase in bulk of this food in the stomach due to absorption of water

The Eat More Index (EMI) Table

The Eat More Index is based on the number of pounds of food it takes to provide 2500 calories. Percent fat by calories are also listed.

FOOD	EMI	FAT%
Scallop	4.88	11
Seaweed (konbu)	12.72	10
Seaweed (wakame)	12.12	11
Sesame	0.94	83
Shrimp	4.75	8
Shrimp, Fried	2.25	46
Soybean	4.20	40
Soybean, sprouts	11.88	28
Spaghetti	4.83	3
Spinach	21.01	11
Squash	28.75	5
Strawberries	14.77	12
Sturgeon	3.41	32
Sugar	1.46	0
Sunflower seeds	0.98	76
Sweet potato	5.36	3
Tangerines	16.07	4
Tofu	7.59	53
Tomato	27.32	8
Tomato paste	6.51	8
Tuna, in water	4.30	17
Tuna sandwich	2.06	46
Tuna, in oil	1.90	64
Turkey	2.08	56
Turkey sandwich	2.13	41
Turnip	19.51	7
Veal	3.44	61
Walnut	0.87	85
Watercress	27.32	13
Watermelon	21.01	7
Yam	6.28	2
Zucchini	32.14	6

APPENDIX III

EXERCISE TABLE

ACTIVITY	Kcal/15 min.
Aerobics (heavy)	146
Aerobics (medium)	91
Back-packing	164
Badminton	99
Basketball (nonvigorous)	173
Basketball (vigorous)	201
Bicycling (6mph)	64
Bicycling (10mph)	100
Bicycling (12mph)	137
Bowling	71
Calisthenics (heavy)	146
Calisthenics (light)	73
Canoeing (2.5mph)	60
Climbing, Mountain	183
Cooking	47
Disco Dancing	110
Football, Touch	137
Gardening	58
Golf (carring clubs)	91
Golf (pull cart)	66
Handball (vigorous)	183
Hiking (cross country)	100
Hiking, Mountain	137
Housework	73
Ice Hockey (vigorous)	183

ACTIVITY	Kcal/15 min.
Ice Skating (10mph)	106
Jazzercise (heavy)	146
Jazzercise (light)	55
Jazzercise (medium)	91
Jog (10min/ mile)	183
Jog (12min/ mile)	155
Jog (13min/ mile)	128
Jog (14min/ mile)	110
Jog (15min/ mile)	91
Jog (17min/ mile)	73
Jog (9min/ mile)	201
Lawn Mowing (hand)	119
Lawn Mowing (power)	66
Racquetball (social)	155
Racquetball (vigorous)	183
Roller Skating	93
Run (5min/mile)	329
Run (6min/mile)	283
Run (7min/mile)	246
Run (8min/mile)	219
Skiing, Cross Country	183
Skiing, Downhill	146
Square Dancing	110
Swimming (fast)	172
Swimming (slow)	141
Tennis, Doubles	91
Tennis, Singles	119
Tennis (vigorous)	155
Volleyball	93
Walking (20min/mile)	64
Walking (26min/mile)	55
Water Skiing	128
Weightlifting (heavy)	164
Weightlifting (light)	73